IF YOUR WORK KEEPS YOU FROM KEEPING IN SHAPE—HERE'S THE BOOK FOR YOU!

YOGA FOR PHYSICAL FITNESS

Written by the nationally famous TV Yoga instructor, Richard Hittleman, YOGA FOR PHYSICAL FITNESS is especially designed for everyone who needs more muscle tone, better circulation and a greater feeling of vitality and well-being.

Over 250 photos geared to 58 simple, effective Yoga techniques make achieving new health—both mentally and physically—easy and fun to do.

All over America, more and more people are turning to Yoga as a way to increase energy and decrease tension. This book can work these wonders for you!

D1208178

ALSO BY RICHARD L. HITTLEMAN

Be Young With Yoga

Yoga For Personal Living

ATTENTION: SCHOOLS AND CORPORATIONS

WARNER books are available at quantity discounts with bulk purchase for educational, business, or sales promotional use. For information, please write to: SPECIAL SALES DEPARTMENT, WARNER BOOKS, 75 ROCKEFELLER PLAZA, NEW YORK, N.Y. 10019

**ARE THERE WARNER BOOKS
YOU WANT BUT CANNOT FIND IN YOUR LOCAL STORES?**

You can get any WARNER BOOKS title in print. Simply send title and retail price, plus 50¢ per order and 10¢ per copy to cover mailing and handling costs for each book desired. New York State and California residents add applicable sales tax. Enclose check or money order only, no cash please, to: WARNER BOOKS, P.O. BOX 690, NEW YORK, N.Y. 10019

YOGA FOR PHYSICAL FITNESS

Richard L. Hittleman

WARNER BOOKS

A Warner Communications Company

WARNER BOOKS EDITION

Copyright © 1964 by Richard L. Hittleman
Copyright under International and Pan-American Copyright
Conventions.

All rights reserved, including the right to reproduce this book,
or any portions thereof, in any form except for the inclusion
of brief quotations in a review.

ISBN 0-446-91281-6

This Warner Books Edition is published by
arrangement with Prentice-Hall, Inc.

Cover photograph by Jerry West

Warner Books, Inc., 75 Rockefeller Plaza, New York, N.Y. 10019

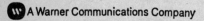 A Warner Communications Company

Printed in the United States of America

Not associated with Warner Press, Inc. of Anderson, Indiana

First Printing: December, 1967

Reissued: May, 1974

20   19   18   17   16   15   14   13

To My Mother and Father

Foreword

No person who is professionally involved in any aspect of maintaining health and physical fitness can doubt the genuine need for a realistic national program for physical fitness. Based on disturbing statistics of general poor health gathered by various state and national health agencies, it now seems the opinion of physicians, physical education instructors and other authorities that some sensible program for physical fitness must be initiated on a national scale. The Federal Government, well aware of the problem, has taken certain preliminary steps in this direction. However, it is the contention of the author that there is a serious error in the concept of the physical fitness program as it is currently being outlined and that unless this error is rectified the program cannot possibly succeed in its *national* intent.

The basic mistake which has been made is to promote the idea of physical fitness in such a way that it has become associated in the minds of most people with *vigorous activities*, the emphasis being on the usual wearisome calisthenics, body building through jumping and running, the use of weights, hikes, sports. Because physical fitness is now associated with these types of activities, *the majority of our population has physically and psychologically excluded itself from the entire idea!*

The truth of the matter is that only a relatively small segment of the population will exercise with calisthenics for more than a short period of time (especially without constant supervision), because this type of exercising is tiring and simply not enjoyable. An infinitesimal number of people will consider conditioning themselves with the use of weights or through regular running and hiking. The people who play tennis, swim, bowl, golf, play basketball, baseball, football, etc., have been doing these things in the past, enjoy them and will in all probability continue to do them without having to be encouraged. But only relatively few people indulge regularly even in these sports. Furthermore, it should be noted that we cannot properly consider weekly or bi-weekly participation in bowling, tennis, golf, etc. to be a method of truly remaining fit. The truth of this statement will be evident as we proceed.

For a national physical fitness program to be of real value, it must be sufficiently comprehensive to include all segments of the population regardless of age, background or vocation, and must help to condition all systems of the body, i.e. not only the muscular and the circulatory, but the respiratory, nervous, endocrine and other aspects of the organism. In addition, such a program must be enjoyable and stimulating so that one wants to exercise if for no other reason than that he feels a sense of well-being after exercising, not exhausted or strained as is so often the case with calisthenics.

The system which meets all of the above requirements is that group of age-old physical movements and exercises comprising the system of Yoga.

In my book *Be Young with Yoga* ° I have explained in detail how the Yoga techniques can be used by everyone to deal with the premature symptoms of "aging." It is the purpose of this book to now offer 58 wonderful Yoga techniques for two groups of people who are in great need of maintaining physical fitness: the *Sedentary Worker* and the *Housewife*. The various routines of Yoga exercises which are offered can

---

° *Be Young with Yoga* (Englewood Cliffs, N.J.: Prentice-Hall, Inc.), 1962.

easily be modified and extended to apply to every segment of the population from the elementary school student to the senior citizen.

One need only give the Yoga system a fair trial, according to the instructions herein, to realize that it can indeed constitute the perfect National Physical Fitness Program.

Los Angeles, California
January, 1964

Models for the photographs are:

Miss Karen Kanell, secretary
Diane Stuart Hittleman, housewife
Richard L. Hittleman

All photographs by *Leonard* of Hollywood except those otherwise credited in the text.

Contents

PART III

SPECIAL PROBLEMS   157

PART IV

YOGA FOR THE HOUSEWIFE 209

PART V

ADVANCED POSITIONS 233

PART VI

PRACTICE ROUTINES: GENERAL INFORMATION 247

Part One

The Sedentary Worker:

Work without Workout

If we were to single out the individual most in need of a program to remain physically fit and least inclined to undertake the exercise necessary to do so, we would have to point to that person referred to as the "sedentary worker." For our purposes in this book, the sedentary worker is: (*a*) the person who is confined to a desk during most of the workday, (*b*) the person whose work is performed in relatively few positions (such as a dentist or a classroom teacher), or (*c*) the person whose work consists of a limited number of repetitious movements (such as a machine operator or a driver).

The major physical fitness problem of the sedentary worker is obvious: He simply does not engage in sufficient *proper* physical activity during the workday. He does not have the opportunity to manipulate his body so that he may prevent such premature characteristics of aging as stiffness, loss of muscle tone, poor circulation and lack of vitality. The problem is compounded by the fact that the usual schedule of the sedentary worker—the time allotted between arising and leaving for work, between the end of the workday and dinner, the family activities in the evening hours—does not seem to allow the time for exercise. If you ask any wholesome, red-blooded American office worker what time of the day he sets aside for his exercise, his eyes will widen with simultaneous contempt and disbelief as he exclaims, "Who has time to exercise?"

Lack of time is the standard excuse. But as already pointed out, the real reason that the sedentary worker does not exercise is because he is mentally and physically "all in" from the day's work, and since the thought of exercising is associated in his mind with jumping and leaping about, it is only natural that he is slightly less than anxious to become more exhausted than he already feels. Ironically, his fatigue, ill-humor or lack of vitality is very possibly due to the stiffness in his back, arms and legs, his poor circulation and those very things which result from the lack of exercise!

We all know that there is always enough time and energy to devote to what we really enjoy, especially if it is beneficial, can be done easily (and in a short period of time if necessary) and requires no special equipment or facilities. This is exactly what Yoga offers us. In Yoga are included enjoyable, nonstrenuous, revitalizing exercises that require a minimum of time and can be done not only before and after the workday but also *during* the workday—in the office, during lunch hour or even the coffee break!

The Back and Spine

The most frequent physical complaints among sedentary workers concern the various areas of the back and spine. If the sedentary worker will stop and think about the movements typical of most of his workday, he will quickly realize that his back is confined to a very few positions and in many cases is actually held "frozen" in one position for prolonged periods of time (especially true of the desk worker). Of course such rigid positions will result in stress. In many cases the positions assumed by the worker, such as those of the dentist or file clerk, place continual pressure on delicate areas of the back and spine, creating a great strain. And even in sitting, the posture assumed by so many desk workers is poor and results in a great deal of discomfort. It is interesting to note that this discomfort has a delayed reaction—often the worker is not aware of how much stress has actually been accumulated until several hours after he has left his office!

Anyone who has ever examined the structure of the back and spine can readily understand why stiffness, tension and cramps occur so easily. The back must have frequent manipulation during the day. The spine must stretch often during the day (something animals well know). Since this manipulation and stretching do not take place during the workday it is essential that they be done after and/or before work. Also, a minute or two for stretching during lunch hour or a break can work wonders, as we shall see.

A surprising number of workers suffer from *constant* back discomfort. Many simply accept this and resign themselves to live with it. Others resort to adjustments, massages, steam, plasters, braces and so forth—all of which have their place and generally offer some relief. However, what is really needed is daily, methodical self-manipulation to loosen cramps and stiffness gradually and to strengthen the weak areas of the back. Strengthening offers the worker an excellent chance of preventing further back aches and pains. He should also be equipped with the knowledge of certain simple, nonstrenuous movements he can perform if and when the back discomforts do arise. How many millions of man-hours of work, representing substantial income for both employee and employer, are lost because of back troubles! How many of these hours could be saved were the worker to apply the Yoga techniques presented in this book!

One who suffers from a major disorder of the back should always receive the permission of his physician before doing any type of exercise. It has been my experience, however, that the mildness of the Yoga movements will meet the approval of almost all physicians. When practicing the Yoga exercises for a particular back problem, you must proceed with caution and not be deceived by the apparent simplicity of many of the movements. The postures are extremely powerful. You will feel how certain exercises effect the lumbar, middle or upper areas of the back. Particular exercises can then be emphasized as needed.

A classic Yoga axiom is well worth your consideration: "You are as young as your spine is flexible." The spine is a "key" to our entire organism. It acts as a communications system and controls many functions of the body and mind. It is able to release energy within the body and promote alertness and clarity of the brain. The science of chiropractic is based almost entirely on the methodical manipulation of the spine. For many centuries the Yogi has stated that the spine must remain supple and flexible throughout life if one is to experience true health. A stiffening spine is a sign of approaching old age, regardless of years, whereas a flexible, supple spine is a major characteristic of youth. (For a detailed discussion of the characteristics of youth see my book *Be Young with Yoga.**) Children have elastic spines, but as they grow older and fail to properly exercise, the spine gradually loses resilience. *There is no natural reason for this to occur.* I have proved to hundreds of thousands of people, through my books, classes and television programs that they can regain the youthful flexibility of the spine practically regardless of age or physical condition. Many Yoga students who are so-called "senior citizens" possess greater flexibility than their grandchildren!

The response of the spine to the Yoga stretching movements is astonishingly quick; it is like a jack-in-the-box that has been compressed into a small area (with the vertebrae often pressing against each other) and is capable of great elongation when the box is opened. The Yoga exercises open the box. Most people are amazed that they can accomplish so many advanced stretching movements within a few weeks of the time they begin their practice, especially since they have grave doubts about their ability when they first see other students performing the movements. As you look through the photographs in this book you may find yourself saying, "I'll never be able to do that." How often I've heard that expression! But reserve your opinions for several weeks. Nature is with you, not against you, when you practice Yoga, and Nature wants your spine to be flexible, not stiff!

Because an important Yoga premise holds that a great amount of untapped energy lies asleep within the spine, many Yoga exercises (*asanas*) are designed to awaken this dormant energy and make it available to the organism. You shall be able to determine the truth of this theory for yourself by practicing the five Yoga exercises that follow.

---

* Richard L. Hittleman, *Be Young with Yoga* (Englewood Cliffs, N.J.: Prentice-Hall, Inc., 1962).

PRELIMINARY LEG PULL

Fig. 1 Sit with your legs stretched straight out before you. The feet should be together. Sit erect but relaxed. Rest your hands on your knees.

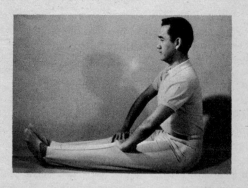

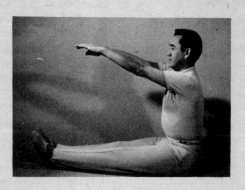

Fig. 2 Slowly and gracefully raise your arms as illustrated.

Fig. 3 Bring your arms up and lean backward several inches. This movement helps to strengthen the abdominal muscles.

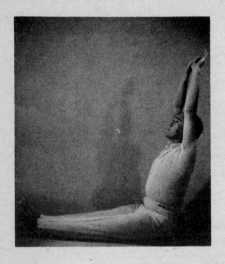

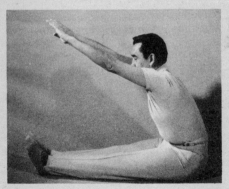

Fig. 4 Slowly and gracefully bring your arms over and lean forward.

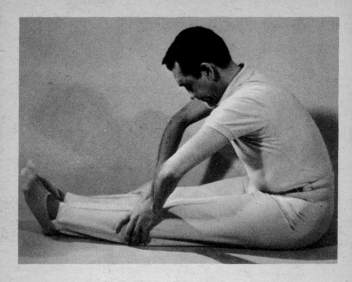

Fig. 5 Take a firm hold on your knees or calves.

Fig. 6 Gently pull your trunk downward as far as you can without strain. Let your elbows bend outward. Let your neck go limp. Hold this position without moving for a count of 5.

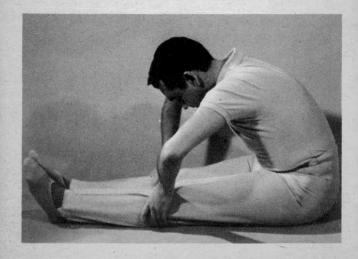

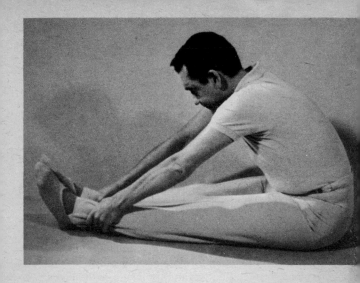

Fig. 7 Slide your hands farther down the legs and attempt to hold the ankles firmly.

Fig. 8 Gently pull your trunk downward as before, bending the elbows outward. Rest your forehead close to your knees if possible. Relax the muscles as much as possible. Do not allow the body to become tense. Hold this position without moving for a count of 5.

Slowly straighten up into the position of *Fig. 1* and repeat both the knee and ankle stretches. Perform three times in all.

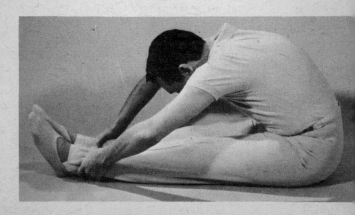

ACTION AND BENEFITS OF THE PRELIMINARY LEG PULL

An absolute must for the sedentary worker, regardless of his field, is to have the ability truly to relax his physical organism for at least several hours after the workday. I use the word *truly* because, to most people, relaxation is synonymous with collapsing into a chair or couch. This, actually the result of fatigue, is not relaxation. Relaxing is an art; it is not inertia and it is not laziness. The cat is the perfect example of a creature who is simultaneously relaxing and building energy (revitalizing).

To learn the lost art of relaxation one must first be able to banish all tension from the body. We are all aware that tension causes nervousness, strain, irritation, weakness and fatigue. It is certain that one of our greatest problems is the inability to relax—physically, emotionally and mentally. But these three aspects of our being are so highly interrelated that what affects one has a corresponding effect on the others. You may be very pleasantly surprised to learn that if you can relax physically you simultaneously achieve a high degree of emotional and mental calm. The Yoga stretching and breathing exercises will remove tension.

The Preliminary Leg Pull provides a good indication of how stiff you may be throughout your legs and spine. Just this simple stretching movement will go a long way toward beginning to loosen these stiff areas. Although you probably know of many stiff and tense points in your body, you are unaware of dozens of other tension areas. Yoga movements, such as the Preliminary Leg Pull, will show up many of these spots.

In the Preliminary Leg Pull, the object is not to see how fast you can fight your way down toward your knees but simply to hold the furthermost area of your legs that you can without strain and pull yourself forward and down easily, so that your spine begins to loosen. The stiffer you find yourself, the greater your need for these gentle pulling movements. Never strain or jerk in these exercises as one is inclined to do in the ordinary type of calisthenics. Just attain your extreme position, regardless of where it may be, and have the patience to hold for a count of 10 and to repeat as indicated. There is no trick to attaining the more extreme position of the Preliminary Leg Pull or, for that matter, of any of the Yoga stretching exercises. It can be achieved when the spine becomes sufficiently flexible.

The Preliminary Leg Pull is a very fine morning exercise that the sedentary worker would find most valuable to practice before leaving for work. This is because the spine is exceptionally stiff in the morning (quite natural after the night's sleep). We have already stated that fatigue and sluggishness can certainly result from a stiff spine, therefore, a few quick movements of the Preliminary Leg Pull are beneficial in loosening the spine. Although these movements will seem particularly difficult in the morning, do not be discouraged—they are of great value. Remember to bend your elbows outward when pulling forward because this enables you to pull more effectively. Also remember to drop your head *downward* when pulling forward, since this helps to work out your neck and upper back muscles. Attempt to remain tranquil and relaxed while performing the movements. Close your eyes in the extreme positions and concentrate on the "feel" of the stretching.

It is important to note that progress in Yoga is irregular. That is, you will find that you can accomplish an extreme position fairly comfortably one day, but that two or three days of practice may be needed before you can do this again. This is the learning process; it is true of almost all Yoga exercises. There are days when you experience what appears to be a setback. I say "appears" because it is not truly a setback. The body is stiff on certain days and does not respond to your will as well as on previous days. But it is really setting itself and preparing to make another stride forward. This is similar to the arrow, which is first pulled *back* before it leaves the bow. This pulling-back movement provides greater impetus to fly forward. When you seem to be having difficulty, your body is drawing itself back like the arrow. If you just "go easy" when you feel stiff and do not force your body or become discouraged, you will find that within a day or two your organism has completed its process of setting and then will take a big step ahead.

COBRA

Fig. 9   Lie with the forehead resting on the floor and the arms at your sides. Relax your body completely. Give in to the floor.

Fig. 10   In slow motion, tilt your head back and using your back muscles, raise your trunk as far from the floor as possible without the use of your hands.

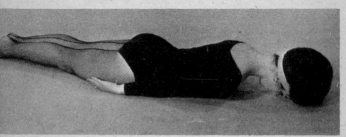

Fig. 9

Fig. 10

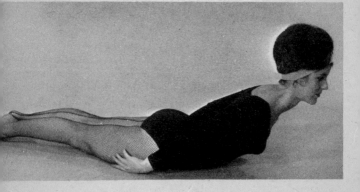

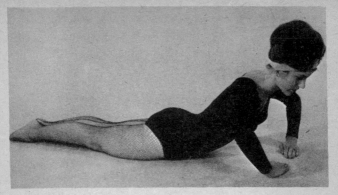

Fig. 11

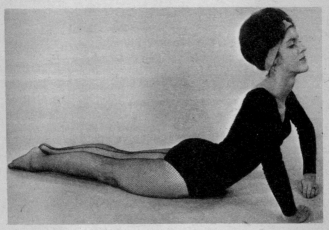

Fig. 12

Fig. 11 Bring in your hands and place them exactly as illustrated—beneath the shoulders with the fingers pointing toward one another.

Fig. 12 Now use your hands to push up very slowly. This pushing up should be done so slowly that you can almost feel each vertebra working out. The head tilts backward, and *the spine is continually arched.*

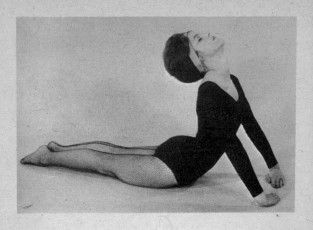

Fig. 13 This is the extreme position of the Cobra. In the beginning you push up only as far as you can without strain, then stop. In this extreme position the arms are straight and the head is tilted far back. The legs are relaxed, not tensed. The eyes may be closed. Hold whatever extreme position you attain for a count of 10.

Fig. 14 Begin to lower yourself very slowly in the exact reverse manner. It is important to keep your spine arched as you come down.

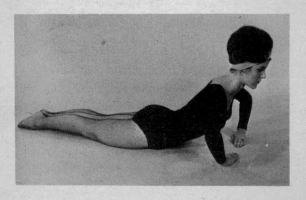

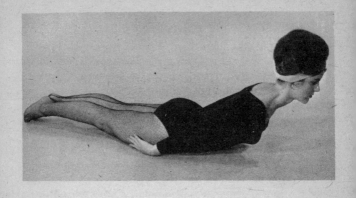

Fig. 15 When you have lowered yourself approximately halfway, bring your arms back to your sides and make your back muscles work.

Fig. 16 When your forehead touches the floor, remain in that position for a few moments, then rest your cheek on the floor. Allow your body to go completely limp.

Perform the entire exercise very slowly twice.

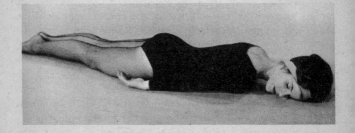

ACTION AND BENEFITS OF THE COBRA

The Cobra is a wonderful series of movements for relieving tension and stiffness throughout the back and spine at any time during the day. Those who have their own offices can take a minute or two and perform the Cobra to loosen the back whenever necessary. Those who have had vertebrae and disc trouble have attained excellent results by utilizing the Cobra movements. While performing the Cobra, you will realize that it is capable of separating vertebrae that may be pushing upon one another. You will also be aware of its strengthening effect upon the discs and the entire back, especially the lumbar area. It is important to remember to keep the head tilted backward throughout the entire exercise. This fine movement for the neck also helps to make certain that the neck muscles and the cervical vertebrae are brought into play.

To gain the full benefits of the Cobra you must also remember that this is not a stiff-back push-up. The spine must continually *arch*. The arching relieves the tension. In the beginning, one should not try to raise himself to the extreme position of *Fig. 13*. He should go only as far as is comfortable and hold that position for the count of 10. Raise yourself a little higher each day. Within a period of about two weeks from the time you begin you should be able to attain the extreme position without strain.

Remember that the Cobra, like so many Yoga postures, is a stretching movement. As such, you should allow your body to remain relaxed whenever possible. In the extreme position practically no muscular effort is needed, so the body, and especially the legs, can relax. The movement in which the trunk is first raised and then lowered without the support of the arms will greatly tone the muscles of the lower back and abdomen. Flabbiness in the hips and buttocks can be considerably reduced through this and certain other Yoga movements you will learn. Note that the movement of the spine in the Cobra is the reverse of that of the preceding exercise. In the Preliminary Leg Pull the spine curved slowly *outward*. In the Cobra, it is curved slowly *inward*.

The Cobra is one of the primary exercises which has enabled many sedentary workers to regain the flexibility of a youthful spine. It is an exercise that should definitely be performed by the worker between his arrival home after work and his dinner. It often prevents the intense letdown period that follows dinner.

BOW

Fig. 17   Lie with your chin resting on the floor and your arms at your sides.

Fig. 18   Bend your legs at the knees and bring the heels in. Reach back and attempt to hold your feet with your hands.

Fig. 17

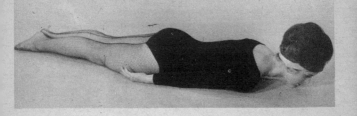

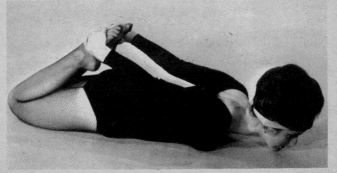

Fig. 18

Fig. 19 Hold your feet firmly and slowly and easily raise your trunk from the floor. Keep your head high. This is the Modified Bow position.

Fig. 20 Keeping the trunk raised, attempt to bring up your knees. Hold your head back. Breathe normally. Hold your extreme position without motion while you count 10.

Fig. 21 It is important to follow these directions for coming out of the Bow. First, lower your knees to the floor but do not let go of your feet.

Fig. 22 Still holding the feet, allow your trunk to be lowered slowly until your chin touches the floor.

Fig. 23 Now release your feet and lower them to the floor. Once they touch the floor, rest your cheek on the floor and allow your body to go completely limp.

Perform the Bow twice.

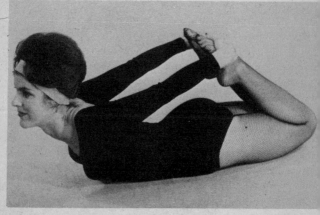

Fig. 19

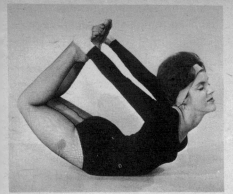

Fig. 20

Fig. 21

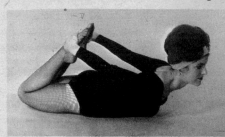

Fig. 22

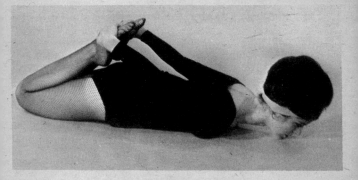

Fig. 23

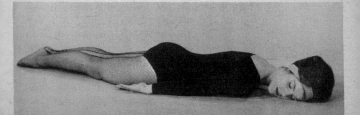

ACTION AND BENEFITS OF THE BOW

The Bow is an extremely powerful movement for building muscle tone and strengthening the entire back and spine. At first, some people have difficulty in reaching back and holding both feet. This can almost always be accomplished after a few tries. If not, a small towel can be held in the hand and looped over the foot. You can see that by holding your feet as described you have a very strong lock against which you pull the trunk upward. In the beginning you must raise the trunk only as far as is possible without strain. This may be only a few inches from the floor. As you continue to practice this movement, the necessary muscular patterns are developed and you can raise the trunk gradually higher. The raising of the knees to complete the posture is, of course, the most difficult part of the exercise. It often takes several months to accomplish this extreme position. But remember that the continual practice is important, not the extreme position. Some feel that if they cannot execute the extreme position of a posture immediately, the exercise is not worth doing. This, of course, is a serious error, since the value is in practicing to improve one's ability.

For the sedentary worker, the Bow is wonderful for toning and strengthening. It develops the chest and bust and is excellent for improving posture.

FULL TWIST

Fig. 24 Sit with your legs extended straight out before you. Now place your right sole firmly against the upper inside of your left thigh.

Fig. 25 Bring in your left foot so that you may hold your left ankle as illustrated.

Fig. 26 Move your left foot over your right knee and place it firmly on the floor.

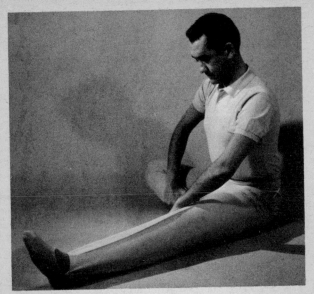
Fig. 24

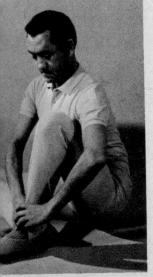
Fig. 25

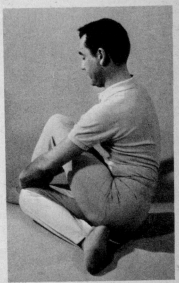
Fig. 26

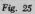

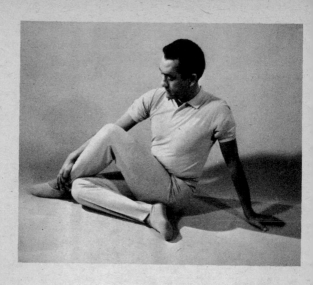

Fig. 27 Place your left hand firmly on the floor behind you.

Fig. 28 Bring your right arm *over* your left leg and hold your right knee firmly.

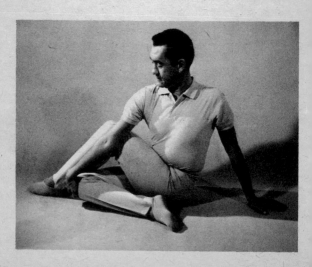

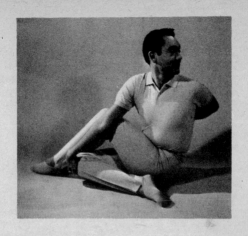

Fig. 29 Slowly twist your trunk and head as far to your *left* as possible. Have your left hand hold the right side of your waist to aid in the twisting movement. Hold this position for a count of 10.

Fig. 30 A back view of the extreme position. Note that the head is turned far to the left and that the hand holds the waist.

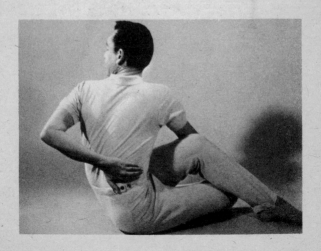

Fig. 31   Return to the frontward position of *Fig. 28*, pause a moment, then repeat the twist. After the second twist, take hold of your left ankle and move the leg back in front of you.

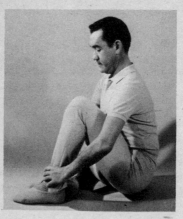

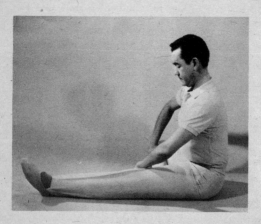

Fig. 32   Stretch out the left leg as illustrated, then the right leg.

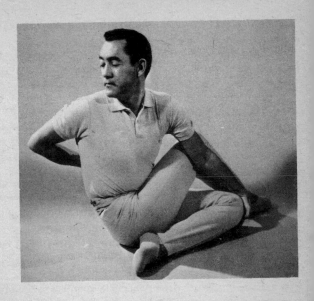

Fig. 33 Perform the identical movements on the opposite side. Substitute the word *left* for *right* in the previous directions. *Fig. 33* depicts the extreme position in twisting to the right.

Perform the Full Twist twice on each side.

ACTION AND BENEFITS OF THE FULL TWIST

There are three basic spinal movements with which we work in our Yoga exercises. The first is the *outward* bending of the spine, as in the Preliminary Leg Pull, the second is the *inward* bending of the spine, as in the Cobra and the Bow, and the third is the spiral *twisting* movement of the Full Twist. In this exercise we can truly see the ingenuity of the Yogi in devising the "locks" and "stretches." In *Fig. 29* the thigh locks the lumbar area of the back so that the middle and upper areas may twist and stretch against this lock. This twisting movement is the quickest spine loosener of any of the Yoga exercises, so the sedentary worker would be wise to learn and practice these positions carefully.

Here are some important tips regarding the exercise: If in *Fig. 26* you have difficulty with your balance when you cross your leg over or if you feel exceptionally cramped in this position, simply push the left leg further away from your right knee. Remember to place your hand down behind you for balance in *Fig. 27*. In *Fig. 28*, note carefully that the arm crosses *over* the left knee—not around or under, but *over*. If you cannot execute this movement comfortably, then follow the suggestion given in connection with *Fig. 26*, that is, push the left leg *away* from the knee. This makes crossing the arm over much easier but lessens the intensity of the lock. Actually, the tighter the lock the greater the benefit. When executing the final position of *Fig. 29* make sure that your head is turned as far to the side as possible. This is important to complete the spiral movement and bring the cervical vertebrae into the exercise. In *Fig. 30* you can see the detail of how the hand holds the waist and aids in the twist. After you have counted to 10 in this extreme position, simply drop your hand back on the floor behind you, turn frontward and rest a moment, then repeat the twist. It is important that you come out of the position exactly as described in *Figs. 31* and *32*. It would be easy to just let everything go and "collapse" out of the position, but remember that it is our objective in these Yoga postures to perform the entire practice with a great deal of style, grace and poise, so that all of your movements take on the feeling of a dance or ballet.

This wonderful Full Twist exercise may take you a few days to perfect because of the number of movements involved and because it is practically a complete exercise course in itself. Your efforts will be well rewarded, however, since once learned you will use it throughout your life. Instinctively, whenever your back becomes tight and your spine is stiff, you will turn to this exercise for loosening. The Full Twist is a serious posture for practice at home. A more simple twisting movement for use during office hours is presented later in the book.

PLOUGH

Fig. 34 Lie flat on your back, arms at your sides, legs relaxed and limp. Rest for several moments in this position with your eyes closed.

Fig. 35 Put your feet together, toes pointing upward; turn your palms down against the floor. Tense your body, push your hands against the floor and, using your abdominal muscles most, raise your legs stiffly from the floor. Keep your knees straight.

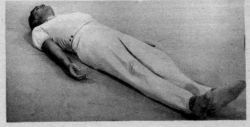

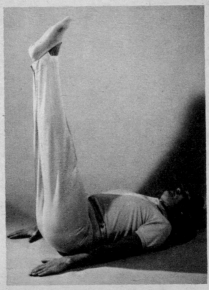

Fig. 36   Bring your legs up all the way so that they make a right angle with the floor.

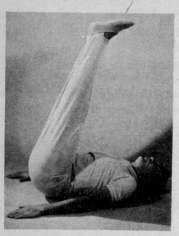

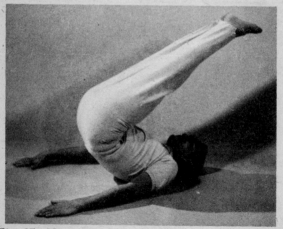

Fig. 37   Now swing your legs back over your head so that the hips are raised from the floor.

Fig. 38 Continue to lower your legs behind you. Keep your knees straight.

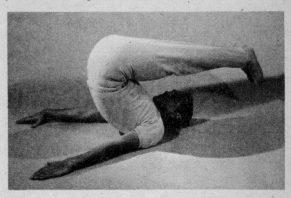

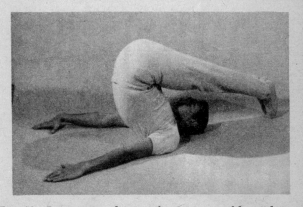

Fig. 39 Lower your legs as far as is possible without strain; stop. The extreme position can be seen in *Fig. 39*, where the toes are touching the floor. The chin will be pressed tightly against the chest. Attempt to breathe normally. Hold whatever extreme position you can attain for a count of 10.

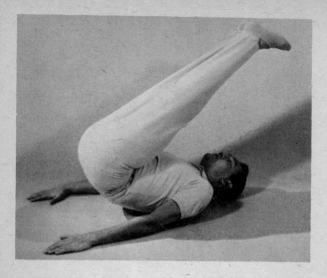

Fig. 40 To come out of the position, bend your knees slightly and begin to roll forward. Arch your neck so that your head can remain on the floor.

Fig. 41 Continue to roll forward and bend your knees until the hips once again touch the floor, as in Fig. 41.

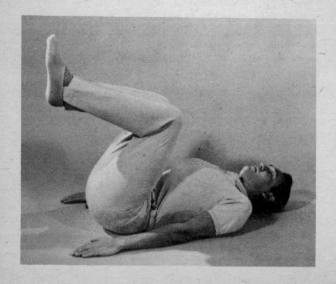

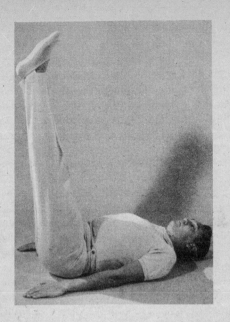

Fig. 42 Now stretch your legs straight upward and lower them very slowly to strengthen the abdominal muscles.

Fig. 43 Rest for a few moments in the position depicted, then repeat the movements. When you have performed the exercise the second time, relax completely and allow your body to go limp, as in *Fig. 34*.

The Plough is performed twice.

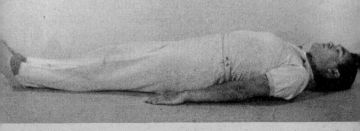

ACTION AND BENEFITS OF THE PLOUGH

In the Plough the vertebrae are bent *outward*, beginning with the base of the spine and progressing upward. You will feel a real sense of accomplishment as your spine gradually "gives," enabling you to touch your feet to the floor in the extreme position. This will indicate that you have gained great elasticity and flexibility. Some find it difficult to raise the hips from the floor, as in *Fig. 37*. This can be due to lack of muscle tone, excess weight and so forth. If the legs are swung backward more quickly, you can generally gain the momentum necessary to raise the trunk from the floor. Once the legs are overhead, it is important to lower them as slowly as possible to permit the vertebrae to be properly worked out. If the legs are lowered quickly, you will not obtain this effect. *Figure 38* represents a modified position of the Plough where the legs have been partially lowered behind you. If you can attain this position within a week or two of practice you are making excellent progress. Remember to keep the knees straight. Gradually, the weight of your legs will stretch your spine so that the feet can touch the floor. Again, there is no trick involved in this exercise; it is simply a question of the spine regaining its natural flexibility. In the extreme position of *Fig. 39*, held for the count of 10, the chin will be pressed against the chest. This may feel awkward or somewhat uncomfortable in the beginning, and normal breathing may be difficult. However, you will find that with a few repetitions the body adjusts itself to the position, and if you concentrate on your breathing you can maintain a regular rhythm.

In coming out of the position it is important to attempt to keep the head on the floor. This can be accomplished by arching the head backward as you roll forward. Otherwise the trunk will come up as you roll forward and you will disrupt the smoothness and grace with which these movements should be performed. In *Fig. 40* you will see how this should be done. *Figures 41* and *42* are primarily for the abdominal muscles. When you perform the movements the second time, the extreme positions will come much more easily.

The Legs

Cramps and pains in the legs are common complaints among
sedentary workers. Due to the usual sitting postures at desks
and many standing postures of the workday, circulation in the
legs grows poor, stiffness sets in and muscle tone is gradually
lost. Most sedentary workers do not do enough walking to
compensate for their long periods of sitting. It should be noted
that the many short walks that some workers take in the office
cannot be considered as true exercise for the legs. This type of
short walking usually leaves the legs much more tired and
strained than exercised.

Here again we find that *stretching* is the best technique for
removing stiffness and cramps. Remember that wherever your
body is stiff, energy is trapped. This is particularly noticeable
with the legs. A worker becomes very tired in the legs although
he uses them very little during the day. Why? Because the
long muscles of the legs grow stiff through inactivity, trapping
energy amidst this stiffness. When we stretch, this trapped
energy is released. The Yoga leg-stretching movements which
follow are most ingenious, since once again they include locks,
and stretches against these locks, enabling you to perform
exactly the amount of stretching that seems necessary. To
work effectively with the legs, longer holding periods are required. In Yoga we prefer to perform only a few repetitions
of most of the exercises placing emphasis on longer holds.

Here are a few tips about the legs that should be of value to the sedentary worker: Circulation is improved if the legs can be raised and rested for a few minutes on a surface several feet from the floor. Executives often do this unconsciously by resting their feet on the desk. This is actually a good practice (except possibly for the surface of the desk). Walking is one of the finest of all forms of exercise because so much of the body is brought into play. A brisk ten-minute walk during lunch hour should be taken whenever possible. Step in a fairly fast, rhythmic tempo. *The steady rhythm is most important in walking.* The arms should swing, and the Yoga Complete Breath (described later in this book) may be practiced simultaneously. This is a most refreshing routine.

Many of the Yoga exercises in this book affect the legs in different ways. The four exercises which follow are very intense stretches, designed for immediate relief of tension, stiffness and cramps. They aid in strengthening, developing and restoring muscle tone. In addition to these four exercises, which are to be done before and after the workday, several leg movements that can be performed within a matter of a few seconds for quick revitalization at any time during the day are presented later in the book.

LEG CLASP

Fig. 44 In a standing position, extend your arms as illustrated.

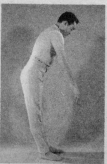

Fig. 45 Bend forward *very slowly* and bring your trunk down as far as possible without straining. Do not bend your knees.

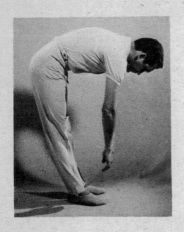

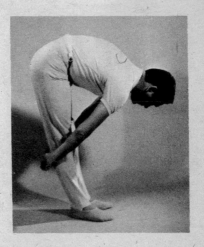

Fig. 46 Clasp your hands behind your knees or calves.

Fig. 47 Very gently pull your trunk as far toward your knees as possible without strain. Hold without moving for a count of 10. After the count is completed allow the trunk to come up slightly but keep the hands clasped. Repeat the stretch.

Fig. 48 Now move the hands as far down the legs as possible and attempt to clasp them at the heels. Pull the trunk forward and gradually try to have the forehead touch the knees. Hold your extreme position for a count of 10. After the count is completed, allow the trunk to come up slightly but keep the hands clasped. Repeat the stretch. Straighten up very slowly after completing the stretches.

Perform the Leg Clasp twice in each of the two positions.

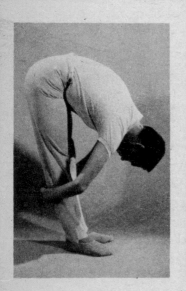
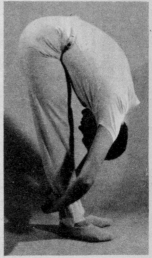

ACTION AND BENEFITS OF THE LEG CLASP

This exercise provides an intensive stretch for the legs (as well as the back) and is excellent for use in the morning when the legs are especially stiff. This may be the only methodical leg stretching the sedentary worker will do throughout the entire day. It certainly is worth taking the one minute necessary to perform the four stretching movements.

This is not the touching-of-the-toes exercise of the well-known 1-2, 1-2 calisthenic rhythm. Such movements can never impart true flexibility to the spine since it is only the quick momentum (which can easily strain the back) that carries the trunk down. If the spine is to gain and retain real flexibility and if the legs are really to stretch, the movements must be done very slowly as described, and the extreme positions must be held. It has been my experience that a sedentary worker will often attempt to prove that he is in excellent physical condition by the fact that he is able to touch his toes. Highly misleading, this indicates nothing except that he has sufficient momentum in his movements to carry his trunk down. If he discontinues his quick, calisthenic movements for several weeks he will become as stiff as a board and have to begin all over again, working for quite some time with his quick movements before he can once again touch his toes. Further, he is always in danger of the back strains that can so easily result from this type of forcing and pulling.

One of the great advantages of Yoga is that once a position is truly mastered you never lose the flexibility or the muscular patterns necessary to perform the exercise, as so many of our older Yoga students well know. That is why we are never in a hurry to attain the extreme positions of any of the Yoga postures. We allow the body to "set" in each of the intermediate positions, and our body itself lets us know when it is ready for the next stage.

In *Fig. 45* we bend forward very slowly and make no attempt to go farther than the body will allow. In *Fig. 46* we clasp the hands at whatever point is comfortable; if we are not able to reach the calves then we hold behind the knees; if we are not able to reach the knees in cases of exceptional stiffness then we hold behind the thighs. The pulling forward in *Fig. 47* is done very gently to allow the spine and legs to stretch slowly and completely. Remember to let the head drop forward. Usually after one or two preliminary stretches it is possible to slide the hands farther down the legs and perform a more intense stretch. Soon your hands should be able to reach the lower calves and then the heels—and this advanced stretch will permit a very great stretch for the tendons and ligaments of the legs. This type of stretching enables you to "become alive" much earlier in the day.

ALTERNATE LEG PULL

Fig. 49 Sit with your legs stretched straight out before you.

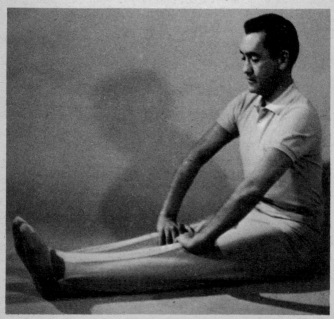

Fig. 50 Place your right heel firmly against the upper inside of your left thigh.

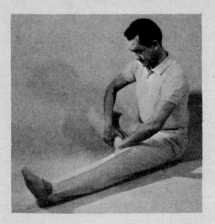

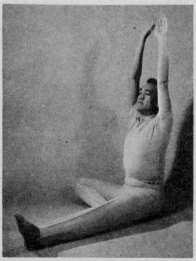

Fig. 51 Reach up and lean backward.

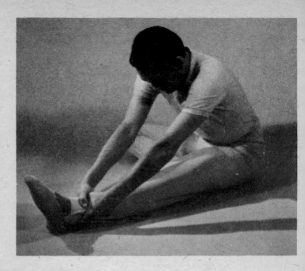

Fig. 52 Bend forward and take a firm hold on your left leg or ankle.

Fig. 53 Gently pull your trunk downward as far as possible without strain. The elbows bend outward. Let your neck go limp. Hold this position without moving for a count of 30. Release the leg, straighten up.

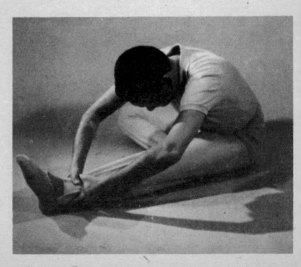

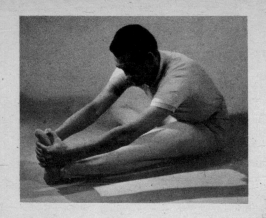

Fig. 54   This is the more advanced position. Reach up and lean backward as in *Fig. 51.* Lean forward slowly and hold the left foot.

Fig. 55   Pull forward. Attempt to have your forehead rest on your left knee. Your elbows bend outward. Hold without moving for a count of 30.

Perform the identical movements with the right leg.

Practice the Alternate Leg Pull twice with each leg. Each position is held for a count of 30.

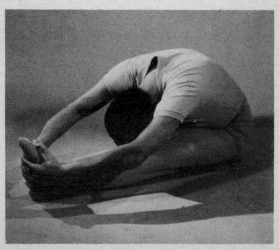

ACTION AND BENEFITS OF THE LEG PULL

The Alternate Leg Pull is the best Yoga exercise for relief of all leg tension. It is a posture which, like the Cobra, should be done upon returning home after work since the stretching revitalizes the legs.

In *Fig. 52*, if for any reason you cannot hold the leg or ankle, simply hold the knee. The back of the knee must always be as close to the floor as possible. It is much better to reach only part way with your arms and keep your leg straight than to reach your ankle or foot by bending your knee. If you bend the knee you will lose the stretch. Naturally, you will feel a great pull in your leg in this posture, and that is exactly what we want. As you gradually work out the stubborn tendons and ligaments of your legs, you will feel more and more comfortable in the Alternate Leg Pull.

Figure 54 represents an advanced position. When you reach forward, bring the foot back toward you to make it easier to grasp. It is important to bend the elbows to aid in the stretch. You can experiment with this by first holding the arms straight, then noticing the much greater pull in the calf when the elbows bend. The knee of *the folded leg* will probably be raised some distance from the floor. This is quite natural in the beginning. As you continue to practice, this knee will drop more and more toward the floor. With steady practice you will soon be able to reach the extreme position and rest your forehead very close to or actually upon your knee. Again, the only trick is sufficient loosening of the spine.

In the beginning you may find it hard to believe that this position is one of the most delightful and restful of all of the postures not only for the legs but for much of the back as well. When you are working with the left leg you will feel a great stretching and firming in the right part of your back. When you are holding the right leg the stretching takes place in the left area of the back. Through these movements you can also help to firm flabby thighs and redistribute excess weight in your legs. We have also found that sedentary workers who have complained of being unable to walk or remain standing for very long without becoming tired in their legs have greatly improved through the practice of the leg pulls.

COMPLETE LEG PULL

Fig. 56 Sit with your legs stretched straight out before you. Always sit erect in these starting positions, and keep your legs together.

Fig. 57 Raise your arms and lean backward as we have already done in several exercises, but now *clasp your hands*.

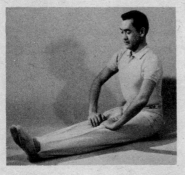

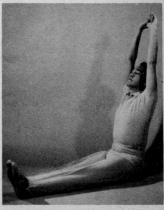

Fig. 58   Begin to come forward very slowly and, as you do, *gently rock from side to side*. Stretch forward as far as possible, keeping your hands clasped.

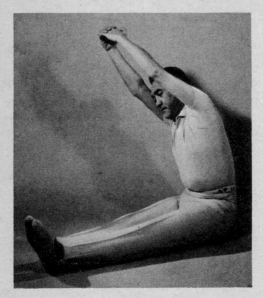

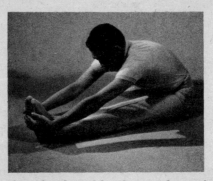

Fig. 59   Place the clasped hands around your feet.

Fig. 60 Bend your elbows, pull your trunk forward and rest your forehead on your knees. Hold your extreme position for a count of 30.

Perform the Complete Leg Pull twice.

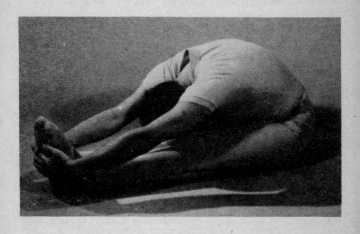

ACTION AND BENEFITS OF THE COMPLETE LEG PULL

This exercise is an advanced position of the Preliminary Leg Pull. The Preliminary Leg Pull places the emphasis on the back, but this exercise is for the legs. For most people the Complete Leg Pull is the most intensive of all of the stretching movements because the longest muscles of the body are involved. You may find yourself quite some distance from being able to hold your feet when you first attempt this exercise but, as already pointed out, the spine is working with you and it will stretch quickly. Almost every Yoga student is able to hold his feet at the end of one month of practice.

There is an important distinction between the last exercise (the Alternate Leg Pull) and this Complete Leg Pull. The Alternate Leg Pull is primarily for relieving tension and revitalizing the legs. The Complete Leg Pull is for developing and strengthening. The rocking motion described in *Fig. 58* is for the purpose of helping to loosen the spine. It is a movement that takes the body very far to the left, then to the right as the trunk comes forward. Bring your feet toward you; this makes the clasping movement easier. If you cannot as yet place the clasped hands around the feet, then separate the hands and simply attempt to hold each foot. The knees must not bend. In the beginning it may only be possible to hold the feet and it may be difficult to achieve much of a stretch. This is perfectly natural, and one should not strain in order to stretch. Simply holding the feet for a count of 30 is sufficient until the spine "gives." It is important to drop your head downward no matter how far forward you can reach. If the head is held stiffly, the neck and upper back do not come into play.

The Complete Leg Pull will go a long way in helping the sedentary worker develop and strengthen the legs without the tiredness, soreness and strain that often follows the once-or-twice-a-week golfing, bowling, tennis or bicycle riding. The legs will also firm evenly through the Complete Leg Pull, without overdevelopment or bulging of the muscles.

ALL FOURS

Fig. 61   Place your body in the position illustrated. Note the position of the toes.

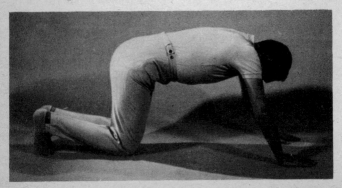

Fig. 62 Without moving your feet, lean forward and slowly raise the entire body as high as possible. Let your neck go limp. Hold this position without motion for a count of 20.

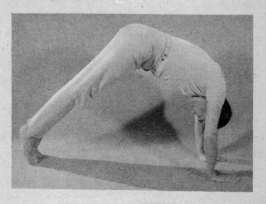

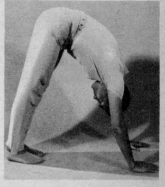

Fig. 63 Move only your feet and walk in toward your head as far as possible without strain. If you can, rest your heels on the floor. Let your neck go limp. Hold this position without motion for a count of 20.

Perform the All Fours exercise twice—once in each position.

ACTION AND BENEFITS OF THE ALL FOURS

This is the last in our series of four Yoga exercises with emphasis on the *entire leg*. In this exercise the legs are stretched, firmed and strengthened in several different positions over which you have complete control. You will be able to feel the various muscles, tendons and ligaments of the legs working out as you assume the two different positions described. In raising the trunk, push up slowly to strengthen the arms. You will find this is also a fine exercise for the muscles of your arms and abdomen.

In *Fig. 63*, attempt to rest your heels on the floor, providing additional stretching for the calves. When you have become comfortable in each of the two positions described, you can attempt an even more advanced position by moving the feet and legs in closer to the head than depicted in *Fig. 63*. This would be quite an extreme position, and the body would resemble a hairpin. The legs would thus receive an extremely intensive stretch.

With a minimum of time and effort, the practice of these four exercises will impart new life to the legs of the sedentary worker—without soreness and strain.

The Knees,
Ankles and Feet

These are real trouble spots for the sedentary worker. They are the points of the body that probably receive less exercise than any other areas, because most people simply do not know how to go about manipulating the knees or the feet. Many, especially those in sedentary occupations, complain relatively early in life of stiffness in the knees and pains and cramps in their feet.

Discomforts that arise from such things as "trick" knees and foot cramps are frequently helped by the Yoga exercises. You will be able to determine the truth of this when you begin to practice the movements of the four exercises which follow. Any point in the knees, ankles, feet or toes where you find yourself growing stiff or inflexible is a danger area, and special attention should be given to working out this stiffness. Even arthritis, as we shall see later, has often responded favorably when these slow, methodical movements are applied.

In attempting to strengthen the feet and remove stiffness from the knees, it is important to place the knees, feet and toes in particular positions and to hold these positions for a prescribed period of time. Many persons are unaware of the different ways in which joints can and should move in order to exercise fully, but the Yoga exercises are most thorough in that they meet both recognized and unrecognized exercising needs by methodically working out the joints and muscles in all possible ways. The same is not true of most sports and forms of calisthenic exercising. If you think about the movements involved in many types of exercising systems and sports, you will realize that the muscles and joints move very erratically in more or less fixed patterns and may thus be strengthened and even overdeveloped in one area but entirely neglected in another. The sedentary worker who states that he gets his exercise by working in his garden on Sunday is fooling himself. He is moving his body more than usual but he is not truly exercising. His back and knees, for example, actually receive a great deal of stress (if he does the usual bending involved in gardening), and he often feels quite tired and strained at the end of the day or upon arising the following morning. He will then think, "I did too much exercising yesterday." Really, he did practically no exercising at all or he would feel revitalized —not fatigued. He has confused *stress* with *exercise*.

During the workday the sedentary worker would benefit considerably if he could take a minute or two to rest his legs in a position in which the *knees bend outward*. Outward bending will loosen the joints and remove tension from the knees. This outward bending simply implies sitting in some form of cross-legged position (approximately as seen in *Fig. 79*) while having lunch or resting in the plant lounge, park and so forth. *Remember, if your knees are stiff your legs will feel tired.*

In this discussion we must also say a word about the torture chambers in which the feet of most workers are encased during the workday. These are known as "shoes." There is no doubt that most shoes have a damaging effect on the feet—hardly news to office workers who rid themselves of their shoes immediately upon coming home. High heels are standard equipment for female office workers, and most men wear a variation of the iron boot. The high heel is deadly in weakening the ankles and cramping the feet. It seems there is little that can currently be done about this situation since in our work we must wear what is required. Of course, special shoes are made for those who must be on their feet a great deal—a matter to investigate as you wish. It is best to walk without shoes as much as possible in your home, and barefoot in your garden, in the country and at the beach. The feet must receive periodic exercise. The exercises that follow can provide this in a matter of minutes.

TOE TWIST

Fig. 64 In a standing position with your feet together, bring your arms up slowly from your sides and simultaneously raise your body to stand on the toes. Allow the hands to touch, and fix your gaze on the back of the hands.

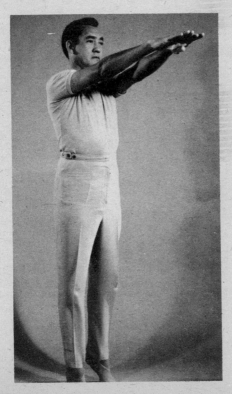

Fig. 65 Remain standing on your toes and *slowly* swing your arms to the left so that your trunk twists at a right angle to your feet. The eyes follow the hands. The feet remain pointing forward and do not change position. Remain on the toes with as little motion as possible for a count of 5. Then return to the frontward position, and lower the arms and legs.

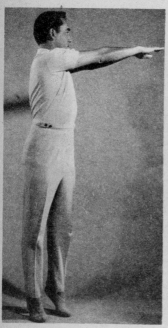 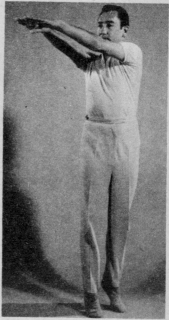

Fig. 66 Slowly perform the identical movements to the right side. Hold for a count of 5 and repeat the movement first to the left and then a second time to the right.

Perform the Toe Twist twice on each side, alternating left and right.

ACTION AND BENEFITS OF THE TOE TWIST

Here we have a fine strengthening movement for the ankles and feet. The exercise requires real control, and there is a great sense of accomplishment in gaining this control. In *Fig. 64*, as you raise onto the toes very slowly, you may get your ankles to "crack," greatly loosening them. It is important that you allow your hands to touch, and that you look only at the back of your hands. In *Fig. 65*, let your arms and hands lead you around to the left. It is most important to make this twisting movement very slowly, since this forces the feet, toes and ankles to work. At first you will continue to lose your balance but, wherever you fall, just pick up your arms again at that very point and continue the twist from there. *Do not laugh at yourself* or become discouraged when you lose your balance. Soon you will gain permanent balance in this exercise. Your carriage and posture will be improved and your confidence in having control of your body will be bolstered. When you have twisted to the extreme position, pull in your abdomen and attempt to stand erect with as little movement as possible while you count 5. Then you turn frontward very slowly, making your feet and legs work and keeping your gaze on the back of your hands. If you lose your balance, pause a moment, regain your composure and come right back up, wherever you are, to continue the movement. When you are facing frontward once again, lower your arms and legs, pause and rest for a few seconds, then perform identical movements to the right.

In this exercise you are asked to gain all the discipline and control of a ballet dancer. Take up the challenge and master these movements. It is easy for the body of the sedentary worker to grow lazy and to feel too tired to stretch or attempt to balance. It is absolutely necessary that the sedentary worker overcome the inertia which will otherwise grow and result in less and less activity. Many people think of their bodies as luggage that is attached to them and that they are forced to carry around. But as they practice Yoga the body is reawakened, and they better understand its significance.

KNEE AND THIGH STRETCH

Fig. 67 Sit erect. Place the soles of your feet together, bring your feet as far in toward you as possible and place your clasped hands around your feet.

Fig. 68 Pull up on your feet and allow your knees to bend gently as far toward the floor as possible. Hold your extreme position for a count of 10. Relax the legs so that they may come upward and rest a few seconds. Repeat.

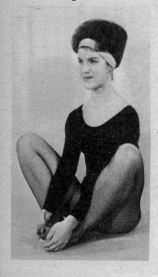

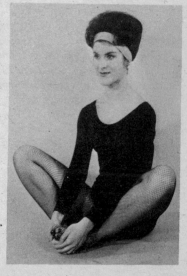

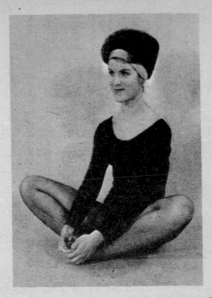

Fig. 69 A more advanced position. Eventually the knees can touch the floor.

Perform the Knee and Thigh Stretch three times.

ACTION AND BENEFITS OF THE KNEE AND THIGH STRETCH

With this exercise for the knees and thighs you can feel the stretched and firmed areas immediately. This movement, which allows the knees and legs to bend outward, is important because it is a stretch seldom performed during the course of an ordinary day's activities. The knees are greatly loosened and the thighs firmed. The physical structures of individuals vary greatly and while some people can place their knees very close to the floor almost at once, most students find themselves quite tight in the muscles, ligaments and tendons of the inside of the legs and thighs. Progress in this exercise is generally slow, but here again it is the practice, not the extreme position, which is important. If the knees will move only a few inches toward the floor the sedentary worker will find this a most delightful feeling because tension is removed and a revitalized sensation follows. Remember to bring the heels in as far as possible and to remain erect throughout the exercise. Do not slump. This exercise is also a very good indication to many people of how tight they have become in certain key areas of the body. Stiffness usually comes as an unpleasant surprise, but the Yoga exercises provide great hope. Remember that no machine, device or gadget can ever truly work out this dangerous stiffness. Only you, through your own methodical movements, can accomplish this.

BACKWARD BEND

Fig. 70 Sit as illustrated. Note the position of the feet and arms.

Fig. 71 Slowly and carefully place your hands on the floor a short distance behind you. The arms should be parallel with your sides and the fingers pointing directly behind you.

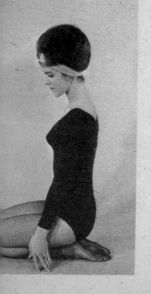
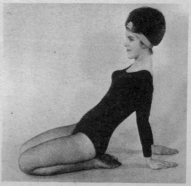

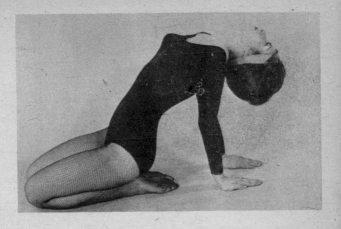

Fig. 72 Arch your back and lower your head. Remain sitting on your heels. Hold without motion for a count of 10. Slowly relax the position.

Fig. 73 Carefully move your hands back as far as possible without strain. Keep your arms parallel with your sides.

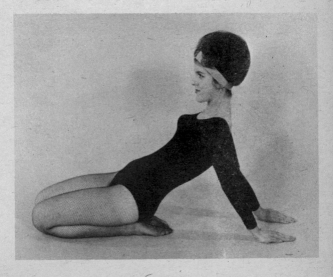

Fig. 74 Arch your back and lower your head. Remain sitting on your heels. Hold without motion for a count of 10. Relax and come forward.

Fig. 75 Change the position of your feet so that the toes rest on the floor and sit as illustrated.

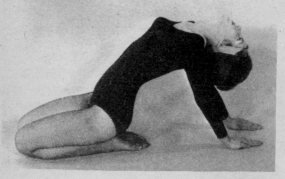

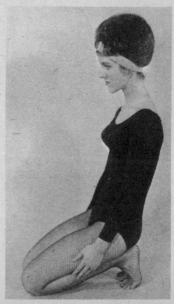

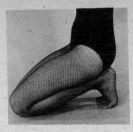

Fig. 76

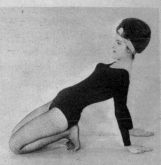

Fig. 77

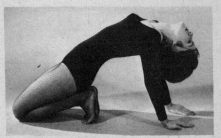

Fig. 78

Fig. 76 A close-up of the sitting position.

Fig. 77 Drop your hands to touch the floor and cautiously inch backward as far as possible without strain.

Fig. 78 Arch your back and lower your head. Remain sitting on your heels. Hold without motion for a count of 10.

Perform the Backward Bend three times—once in each of the three positions.

ACTION AND BENEFITS OF THE BACKWARD BEND

The Backward Bend involves the entire body. From it are derived many wonderful benefits. For our purposes we will emphasize the benefits for the feet and toes. When you sit on your heels, as in *Figs. 70-74,* you stretch and strengthen the feet. Holding the arms parallel as advised is good for the shoulders and for muscle tone in the upper arms. Remember to stay on the heels when you arch your spine (otherwise, you lose the stretch). In *Fig. 74,* the stretch is much greater than in *Fig. 72* because of the increased distance. In *Fig. 75* we undertake the most intensive of all strengthening movements for the feet and toes.

For most sedentary workers, attempting to perform this exercise is conclusive proof of how stiff this area of the body has become. Many find this movement painful, especially if they attempt to rest the full weight of the body on the toes all at once. Usually only a limited amount of the body weight should be placed on the heels in the beginning. Each day the toes will grow a little stronger and will be able to support more weight. Gradually the full weight of the body can rest on the heels. The stretching movement on the toes as shown in *Figs.* 77 and 78 must be done very cautiously to avoid strain. Make sure that you inch backward carefully with your hands. Do not lunge backward. *Figure* 78 depicts a stretch that, due to the increased height of the trunk when the toes rest on the floor, is very great. This is the most intensive movement for the ankles, feet and toes. The more difficult or painful this movement feels at first, the more important that you master it. I have never taught this exercise to anyone who could not accomplish the extreme position within two months of practice.

LOTUS POSTURES

Fig. 79 The simplest of the cross-legged postures. Persons who are exceptionally stiff or overweight must begin limbering up the legs and knees by assuming this position.

Fig. 80 The first movement of the Half-Lotus. The left heel is placed as close to the body as possible, and the sole is against the right thigh.

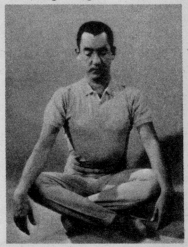

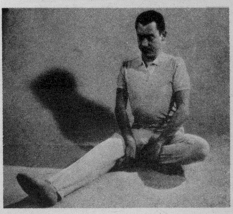

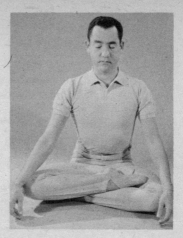

Fig. 81 The right foot is placed on top of the left thigh as illustrated. Carefully note the position of the foot. The heel should be as far in toward the groin as possible. The hands rest easily on the knees. The eyelids are lowered, not closed. This position is assumed for a number of different purposes (to be explained). It can be held as long as is comfortable.

Fig. 82 The first movement of the Full-Lotus. The left foot is placed high on the right thigh.

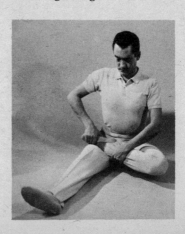

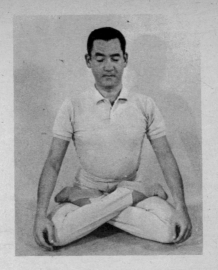

Fig. 83 The completed Full-Lotus. The right foot has been placed high on the left thigh.

Fig. 84 The hands rest on the knees with the index finger of both hands touching the second joint of the thumb. The eyelids are lowered, not closed. This is the full meditation posture.

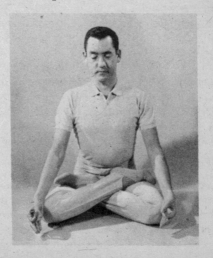

ACTION AND BENEFITS OF THE LOTUS

There are two aspects of the Lotus Postures: one physical and one mental. Physically, it is wonderful for the knees, ankles and feet. No one is expected to accomplish the Full-Lotus upon first attempts (although there are exceptions). Even the Half-Lotus will be difficult for many people. Again, the aim is not to achieve the advanced postures, but to practice methodically the movements that lead toward their mastery. The movement of *Fig. 80* should present no problem. In *Fig. 81* it is desirable to place the left foot as high as possible on the right thigh. If this is difficult, then the foot may be placed lower—on the right calf. You may find your left knee quite high in the air, usually because of the tightness of the muscles and ligaments in the thigh. If you will simply rest your hand or lower arm on the left knee, the thigh will gradually stretch out and the knee will lower itself toward the floor. Make no attempt to push or force the knee down. It will not stay. Only patient sitting will lower the knee. After sitting in this position for about two minutes, the legs should be reversed, that is, the left foot and leg should be placed on the bottom and the right on top. You will quickly feel what a powerful exercise this is for the knees as well as for the ankles.

The Full-Lotus is an advanced posture and is attained through practice. The very best way to practice for the Full-Lotus is to rest with one foot on the thigh as depicted in *Fig. 82*. Once your knee is able to touch the floor without help from the hands you will be able to do the Full-Lotus. As long as the knee is in the air, the opposite leg cannot be placed on top of the thigh—because the moment it is raised the balance is lost. Practice for the Full-Lotus with both legs. Hold the position of *Fig. 82* for one minute, then reverse the legs.

Now as to the mental aspect of the Lotus Postures. These postures are not curiosities nor are they parlor tricks to surprise your friends. They were designed for a profound form of relaxation. As you practice the Lotus Postures you will soon come to realize that these positions represent the most relaxed form of sitting. This is because the legs are literally taken "out of the way"; you do not have to move the legs very frequently as you do when sitting in the usual positions, with the legs hanging down from the chair, bed or couch and blood flowing into them. It is impossible to relax in the real sense of the word when you must change your physical position frequently. It is impossible to meditate when the body must continually move. This is because when the body moves the mind moves. Let us look further into this concept.

It is absolutely essential that the sedentary worker take a few minutes for mental relaxation and rejuvenation after the workday. He must be able to withdraw his mind from the many activities of the day and allow it to rest. This process of resting or, in a sense, "shutting off the mind" is termed *reflection, concentration* or *meditation*. These terms have different meanings for different people, but in general imply a departure from the usual way in which the mind is used during the ordinary day's activities. For many, many centuries the Yogis have taught that the most efficient way of practicing the various forms of meditation is to assume first a physical position in which the body is entirely comfortable while fully awake. The Lotus Postures are the results of painstaking experiments by the great Yogis of the past to perfect the desirable meditation positions.

You may engage in any form of meditation. You may allow your mind to dwell on a pleasant thought or symbol, practice your affirmations or positive thinking, silently chant or pray and so forth. One sits on his mat or cushion in the Half- or Full-Lotus Posture (or, if this is not possible, the simple cross-legged position of *Fig.* 79), places his hands and fingers in the position of *Fig.* 84, keeps the spine erect and lowers the eyelids. The eyes are not closed, because this is associated with sleep. The eyelids are lowered so that a slit of light comes through. The breathing will automatically slow down after a minute or so in the posture. This is also important, because a slowing of the breathing helps to rest the mind. (Quick or

erratic breathing always produces excitement and vice versa.)
The Lotus Posture is held only as long as it is comfortable;
the legs then can be reversed. In the beginning it may be comfortable for only a minute or two, but one can quickly reach
five minutes. These are five minutes extremely well spent in
the interest of the sedentary worker's mental health.

Miscellaneous Techniques
for
Seldom Exercised Areas

The following series of five Yoga techniques is simple, but of great value. It exercises vital areas where the organism of the sedentary worker, so to speak, "goes to sleep." The joints of the elbows and shoulders, (arthritis and bursitis strongholds) are given careful attention and the neck and eyes (places where great tension accumulates) are methodically exercised. Even the scalp, an area not considered in most systems of exercising, is stimulated to promote healthy growth of hair. The entire routine can be practiced within a matter of five minutes!

ELBOW EXERCISE

Fig. 85 This exercise loosens the joints of the elbows. Sitting in a cross-legged position, raise the arms as illustrated. Make two fists of the hands and bend the arms.

Fig. 86 The arms are "snapped" out. It is one of the few quick movements in the system. The elbows will usually "crack" in this movement. Hold the arms straight for a moment. Then bend the arms and repeat the movement.

Perform the Elbow Exercise five times.

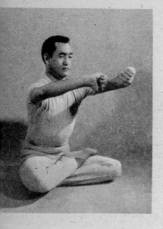

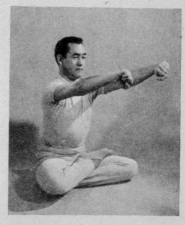

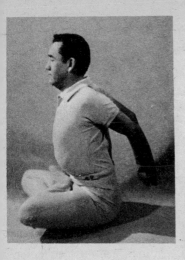

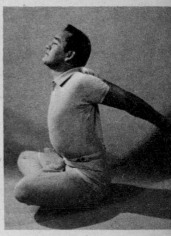

SHOULDER RAISE

Fig. 87 In a cross-legged posture, clasp your hands as illustrated. Keep the spine straight.

Fig. 88 *Very slowly* raise your arms as high as possible without strain. Straighten the elbows if you can. Keep your spine straight. Hold your extreme position without motion for a count of 5. Slowly lower your arms. Repeat.

Perform the Shoulder Raise three times.

Action and Benefits of the Shoulder Raise

Here is a fine, nonstrenuous movement for quick relief of tension in the shoulders and firming the upper arms. The area of the back shoulder muscles is a place where tension accumulates easily, and people who work at a desk are very much aware of this. The positions required for writing and typing cause rounded shoulders and poor posture in general. This results in fatigue because stress is placed on the shoulder and neck muscles. Also, alertness is always diminished when the spine is cramped, as it is with poor postures.

This condition can be greatly helped if the shoulders are frequently brought up and back. The Shoulder Raise provides this movement. You will feel that the upper arms are firmed and flabbiness reduced. In *Fig. 88*, the arms are brought up as far as possible. This will vary with the individual according to stiffness or structure. We try to straighten the elbows, but this is not essential. Remember that the spine must be straight at all times. This is a movement that many desk workers can do in their chairs.

NECK TWIST

Fig. 89 Place your elbows on a level surface (floor, table, desk). Elbows should be fairly close together, arms parallel. Place your head between your hands.

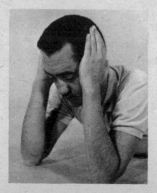

Fig. 90 Clasp your hands on the lower back of your head and gently push down until your chin touches your chest. Close your eyes. Hold for a count of 10.

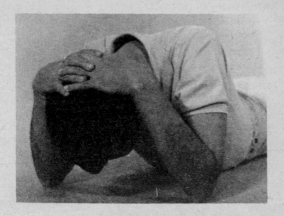

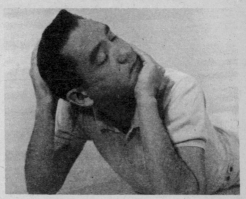

Fig. 91 Do not move your arms. Turn your head *slowly* and rest your chin in your left arm. Grip the back of your head firmly with your right hand. Turn your head *slowly* as far as possible to your left. Keep your eyes closed. Hold your extreme position for a count of 10.

Fig. 92 Do not move your arms. Turn your head *slowly* and rest your chin in your right palm. Grip the back of your head firmly with your left hand. Turn your head *slowly* as far as possible to your right. Keep your eyes closed. Hold your extreme position for a count of 10.

Perform the Neck Twist once in each of the three positions.

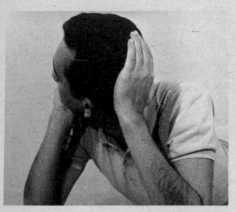

ACTION AND BENEFITS OF THE NECK TWIST

The neck area is most subject to tension, stiffness and general discomfort. This is readily understood when you examine the complex of nerves and muscles in the neck and then consider how rigidly it is held during much of the workday. The sedentary worker will see many of his co-workers utilizing all types of neck-stretching movements to relieve the ever present "stiff neck." These movements usually take the form of quickly rolling the head from side to side in an effort to reach the troubled muscles. But quick movements made in a hit-and-miss fashion cannot give the neck a thorough working out. The Neck Twist exercise, done slowly and methodically, will prove invaluable to the sedentary worker.

The value of the Neck Twist lies in the way the hands are used to manipulate the neck and hold it in the extreme positions. In *Fig. 90*, the hands are clasped on the back part of the head (not the neck) and the head is pushed down so that the back neck muscles and the cervical vertebrae are worked. Make sure your elbows are fairly close together so that you have enough height to move your head downward toward your chest. In *Fig. 91*, it is important that your hands have a good grip on your head so that you can turn it properly. Notice that the chin rests firmly in the hand and that the left fingers are on the left cheek (not the right cheek). The reverse would be true in *Fig. 92*. The head is slowly turned to the side as far as it will go. Without the aid of the hands it could not turn as far (it is this extra inch or two which does so much in loosening and strengthening). Make no attempt to "crack" the neck with any quick, sudden or forceful movements. Simply turn as far as possible and hold for the count of 10. The neck will gradually loosen and you will be able to turn farther to the side. In cases of exceptional stiffness, proceed with great caution; you may hold your extreme position for a count of 25 or even more if necessary. These neck movements usually feel quite delightful as you close your eyes to relax and enjoy the stretch.

EYE EXERCISE

Fig. 93   Widen the eye sockets. Move your eyes to the extreme top of the sockets. Hold one second.

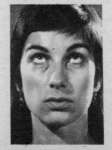

Edward A. Bollinger

Fig. 94 Roll your eyes to the extreme right. Keep the sockets wide open. Hold one second.

Roll your eyes to the extreme bottom. Hold one second.

Roll your eyes to the extreme left. Hold one second.

Perform the Eye Exercise ten times clockwise, ten times counterclockwise.

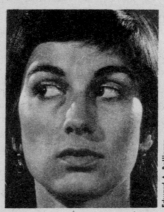

Edward A. Bollinger

ACTION AND BENEFITS OF THE EYE EXERCISE

All sedentary workers need to exercise the muscles of their eyes. They are dependent for their living on their eyes; it is therefore a serious error not to give them whatever care is possible. The Eye Exercise presented here will help to relieve tension that accumulates in the area of the eyes and will help to strengthen the muscles. There are many other eye exercises for different purposes. You may have done various eye exercises in the past. This eye exercise requires less than two minutes to perform the twenty rounds.

Keep the sockets wide. This widening, stretching movement helps to relieve tension around the eyes. Headaches are often due to misuse or overuse of the eyes and to tension that builds up in the eye area. As the eyes are moved to the four positions in this exercise, keep the sockets wide and make sure that the eyes roll to the extreme position so that the muscles really work. Pause in each of the positions for a moment; this is not a continuous roll. When you have completed ten clockwise rounds (moving first to the right), close the eyes and rest them for a few moments. Then open them and perform the counter-clockwise movements (moving first to the extreme left).

The inverted postures, in which the head is down and the flow of the blood into the head is increased, help promote the health of the eyes. The Plough, Shoulder Stand and Head Stand are examples. There are several points that the sedentary worker should consider in connection with his eyes. First, he must always be certain that he has the correct amount of light for his work. He must avoid glare. It is an excellent practice to stop working for a few moments once or twice during the day and "palm" the eyes. That is, remove glasses and place the palms over your eyes so that they rest in complete darkness. This practice helps to relax the eyes. Vitamin A is essential for the health of the eyes. Make sure your diet contains a sufficient amount of this vitamin; the current minimum daily requirements of Vitamin A are set at 5000 international units. A few of the best sources are fresh or cooked carrots, sweet potatoes, beef and calf liver, spinach, turnips, parsley and cod liver oil.

SCALP EXERCISE

Fig. 95 Grasp as much of the hair as possible with your hands.

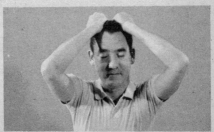

Fig. 96 Pull forward so that the scalp moves. In continuous motion, pull forward and backward, moving the scalp as much as possible.

Perform ten rounds of the Scalp Exercise.

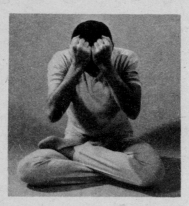

ACTION AND BENEFITS OF THE SCALP EXERCISE

The appearance of the hair is dependent on the condition of the scalp. It is the firm conviction of the Yogi that the best way to maintain both the health of the scalp and fine appearance of the hair is to nourish the scalp by bringing the blood into this area. Inverted Yoga postures such as the Head Stands greatly increase the flow of blood directly into the head and scalp. The Scalp Exercise is designed for stimulation and to keep the scalp from becoming tight. You will find that where hair has fallen out and baldness has occurred, the scalp is rigid. It is therefore reasoned that if the scalp is kept loose one has a better chance of preventing the hair from falling out and of promoting its lustrous appearance.

In *Fig. 95* the hair is grasped very firmly. In *Fig. 96*, don't be too gentle when you pull to and fro. Feel the pull deeply in the scalp. You will find this movement leaves the scalp feeling alive and invigorated.

Blood Circulation

Most of the daily activities of the sedentary worker require him to sit or stand in ways that cause the blood to flow predominantly downward into the lower parts of the body while the organs and glands situated above the heart (especially in the neck and head areas) often do not receive proper circulation. Remember that the heart is always pumping *against* gravity to circulate the blood into the upper areas. This becomes more difficult for your heart as you grow older and become less active. In the sedentary worker poor blood circulation can occur at a relatively early age.

The blood is the life fluid of the body. Every cell in the entire organism is dependent on the blood for its nourishment, for its very life. Not only does the flow of the blood carry the food from which the cells build and repair but it takes away waste products that would otherwise poison your body. If the quality of your blood is high (as a result of proper nutrition) and your circulation good, you are quite certain to feel healthy and alive. If the circulation is poor, the negative consequences are innumerable. Indeed, most people are well aware of these facts, but very few have any knowledge of how to improve their circulation.

The series of Yoga exercises that follow should work wonders for the circulation. If your circulation is good these exercises should keep it so; if you want to improve the appearance of your complexion and your hair these exercises will help. Many major and minor problems that people attempt to treat externally are in reality internal problems, and remarkable improvements (from the stopping of falling hair to better vision and hearing) are noticed when these circulation exercises are undertaken. This series of postures and techniques has two aspects: *breathing* and *inverting the body*. Learning to breathe fully and correctly is essential to improve the quality of the blood as well as to aid circulation. Inverting the body has a direct and immediate effect on circulation. For the sedentary worker the quickest way to restore alertness is to allow the blood to run into the head! With the body in an inverted position, organs and glands that are usually *above* the heart are now *below* it. Thus an increased supply of blood flows into these areas. The effect of this simple maneuver on the entire organism is truly remarkable. That is why we are seeing more and more pictures in newspapers and magazines of statesmen, creative people and executives using the inverted techniques (Head Stand and Shoulder Stand).

Several breathing and inverted techniques can be done *during* the workday to refresh and revitalize within minutes.

COMPLETE BREATH

Fig. 97 Sit in a comfortable cross-legged posture. The Half or Full-Lotus positions are best. Exhale very deeply so that the lungs are emptied of air. Pull in your abdomen as far as possible to help with the exhalation.

Fig. 98 *Begin a very slow inhalation through your nose.* As you inhale, also begin to distend your abdomen.

Fig. 99 Continue the slow inhalation. Now distend your abdomen as far as possible. Make this an exaggerated movement.

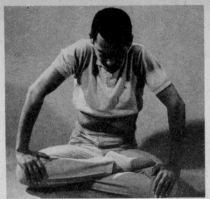

Fig. 97

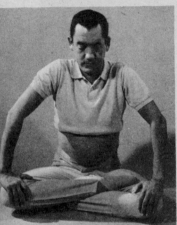

Fig. 98

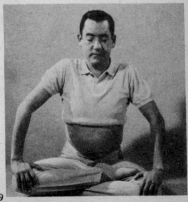

Fig. 99

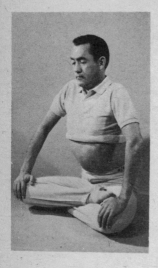

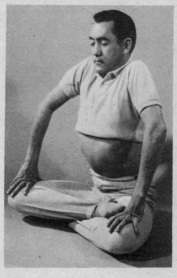

Fig. 100 Continue the slow inhalation. Slowly expand your chest as far as possible. Make this an exaggerated expansion.

Fig. 101 Continue the inhalation. Keep your chest expanded and now raise your shoulders as illustrated. This is the completed posture. Hold for a count of 5.

Very slowly exhale completely through your nose and simultaneously allow your body to contract and relax. Exhale very deeply and, without pause, repeat.

Perform the Complete Breath three times.

ACTION AND BENEFITS OF THE COMPLETE BREATH

Few things can be of more importance to the health of the sedentary worker than some form of breathing exercise that will fill his lungs with air. During office hours the sedentary worker will find that he breathes in a very shallow manner. This usually takes the form of what is known as "high breathing," in which only the upper part of the lungs is used. Consequently, a minimum amount of air enters the lungs. The various sitting and stooped postures of the sedentary worker often cause this limited type of breathing. Very few offices are well ventilated with fresh air. Either they are poorly ventilated and filled with polluted city air and cigarette smoke or they are air-conditioned. An air-conditioned office is certainly far from healthful and has a most negative effect on many workers, causing colds and muscular pains.

Even when most people attempt to take what is referred to as a "deep breath," they use the lungs only partially because they do not know how to utilize the lungs in their entirety. The objective of the Yoga Complete Breath is to enable the sedentary worker to do exactly this. "Life is in the breath," states the Yogi and so it is. He who only half-breathes, half-lives. The lungs enable the heart to function. Man can go for weeks and even months without a scrap of food, but for scarcely three minutes without breath. Alertness and clarity of the mind are directly dependent on the type of breathing one does. All of the foregoing statements should be carefully considered by every office worker. With a little thought and experimentation one will certainly reach the conclusion that the quality of his life, mental and emotional as well as physical, is completely involved with his breathing.

The Yogis have known this since time immemorial. Countless centuries ago they observed the relationship between breathing and the various aspects of physical, emotional and even spiritual development! Breathing forms the basis of Physical (*Hatha*) Yoga, and most of our exercises can be practiced with breathing. This will be discussed in detail. The

Yogis were probably the first group to recognize the effect of certain forms of breathing on the nervous system and to perfect various methods of relaxation through breathing. We shall also learn these.

The Complete Breath is the basic breathing exercise in this course, and the sedentary worker must learn it well. Let us discuss some of the fine points. In order to perform the important body movements of *Figs. 98-101*, it is obviously necessary that the inhalation be a very slow one. You may find it difficult to control your breathing so that you can breathe as slowly as is necessary. If this is the case, then you must practice only the slow inhalation and exhalation until you gain some control. It may take a little time to perfect this slowness, and you may find yourself yawning and becoming impatient. But you must persist in this practice because it is of utmost importance. Once you have gained control of the slow breath it must be combined with the body movements. In *Figs. 98* and *99* you are asked to push out the abdomen and literally form a "big belly." This movement is not difficult and merely requires some control of the abdominal muscles. This pushing out of the abdomen will allow the inhaled air to reach the lower part of the lungs. (The reason that the so-called "deep breath," which in calisthenics takes the form of a quick and noisy snorting in and out, does not reach the lower lungs is because the abdominal area is always pulled in and up.) The next movement is also relatively easy. Expand your ribs to produce a large and exaggerated chest. The final movement of *Fig. 101*, in which the shoulders are raised, allows the air to enter the highest part of the lungs. The position is held for a count of 5 so that the blood can absorb the oxygen. The eyes may remain closed throughout the movements. The exhalation must be as slow as the inhalation but no particular body movements are necessary, except to slowly relax the entire body. The exhalation is very deep, with the abdomen being contracted to force all air from the lungs. Without pause, the next Complete Breath is begun.

Try to have a supply of fresh air coming into your room when you practice the Complete Breath. You can practice a *modified* form of the Complete Breath almost anywhere when necessary to clear your thinking and help in revitalization. It can be done in conjunction with a brisk walk during lunch hour or at other walking periods; it can be practiced in the office. In the Modified Complete Breath, the exaggerated movements are not performed and the last movement of raising the shoulders is eliminated in order to avoid attracting attention. The same slow inhalation is performed and the abdomen and chest are expanded moderately. The benefits of this type of breathing are self-evident and will be noticed almost immediately.

COMPLETE BREATH STANDING

Fig. 102 Stand as illustrated. Exhale deeply.

Fig. 103 Slowly raise the arms as illustrated while simultaneously inhaling and performing the abdominal and chest movements of the Complete Breath as just learned in the previous exercise.

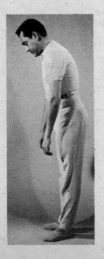
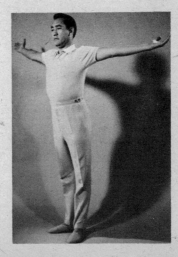

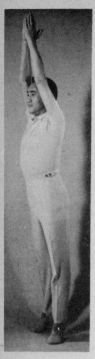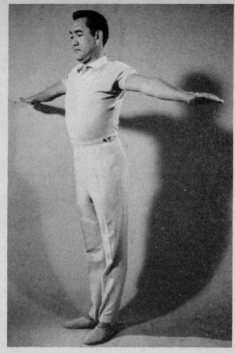

Fig. 104 Continue the inhalation; also continue the raising of the arms until the hands touch overhead as illustrated. Come up on the toes just before the hands touch. The breath is now completed. Hold for a count of 5.

Fig. 105 Slowly exhale and lower the arms. Come down on the soles of the feet.

Fig. 106 Continue a very deep exhalation. The abdomen is contracted entirely and you allow yourself to "wither." The body hangs limp as the deep exhalation is completed. Then the inhalation and body movements are begun again.

Perform the Complete Breath Standing three times.

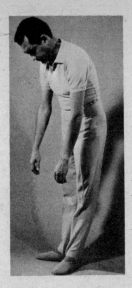

ACTION AND BENEFITS OF THE COMPLETE BREATH STANDING

These movements are more like a dance than an exercise, and you should have the dance attitude in mind as you perform them. This is a highly revitalizing series of movements, since the entire body is involved. In *Fig. 102*, stand in a relaxed fashion, exhale deeply, then begin to inhale slowly while pushing out in the abdominal area. The arms begin to come up with the palms upward, and the chest is also expanded while the inhalation is continued. The completed posture can be seen in *Fig. 104*. The touching of the palms overhead automatically causes the shoulders to be raised, and the breathing is completed at this point. The elbows can be held straight, with the hands in a symmetrical position directly overhead. Standing on the toes (begun when the arms are approximately half-raised) completes the dance-like attitude. In the movements of *Figs. 102-104*, the feeling is one of growing or "blooming," much as you would envision the growth of a flower. In *Figs. 105* and *106* the opposite feeling ("withering") is portrayed through body movements and deep exhalation.

RISHI'S POSTURE

Fig. 107 Stand erect with your feet slightly apart and raise your arms as illustrated. Place the hands together.

Fig. 108 Slowly turn 90 degrees to your left, keeping your eyes on your hands. Only the trunk is turned, not the feet.

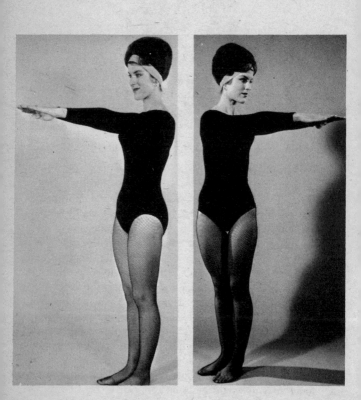

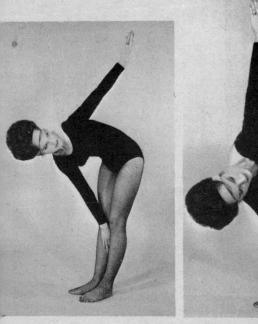
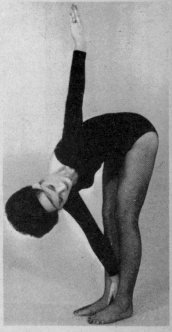

Fig. 109 Look carefully at the illustration. Bend slowly at your waist so that your *right hand* slides down the back of your *right leg* and your eyes look at the back of your left hand.

Fig. 110 The extreme position, in which the right hand is holding the right heel and the eyes look at the left hand directly overhead. The knees are held straight. If this extreme position is too advanced, then simply go as far down as possible and hold your extreme position for a count of 5.

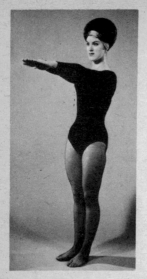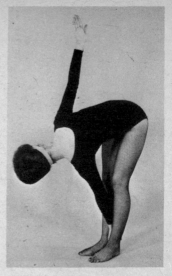

Fig. 111 *Slowly* straighten up, bringing your arms and hands together once again.

Fig. 112 Perform the identical movements on the right side.

Perform the Rishi's Posture twice on each side, alternating the sides.

ACTION AND BENEFITS OF THE RISHI'S POSTURE

This is another of our "dance" postures, in which the movements are performed with grace and poise. The twisting and bending movements are excellent for improving circulation of the blood and promoting flexibility and co-ordination of the body. A *Rishi* in Sanskrit is a great, wise teacher; this particular exercise, however, does not seem to have any obvious connection with the word.

Figure 108 provides a twisting movement similar to the Toe Twist. Keep your eyes on your hands and let them lead you around to the side. Keep your abdomen pulled in. In *Fig. 109*, make certain that your right hand slides down the *inside* and *back* of your right leg (not the outside and not the left leg). You must keep your legs straight (do not bend the knees), and you must at all times be able to see the back of your left hand. If your hand is out of your sight, then you have not yet gained sufficient flexibility and should not lower your trunk so far. *Figure 110* illustrates the extreme posture. You will see the back view of the extreme posture in *Fig. 112*. The body has a beautiful symmetry in these extreme positions, and you may be interested in observing the various geometrical figures formed by the limbs and the trunk. You straighten up slowly from the extreme position, bring the hands together in front, then twist to the right.

SHOULDER STAND

Fig. 113 Lie flat with your arms at your sides, and allow your body to go completely limp.

Fig. 114 Brace your palms firmly against the floor, tense your abdominal and leg muscles and slowly raise your legs as illustrated.

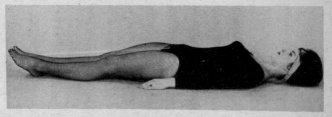

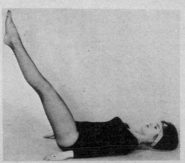

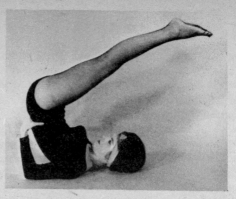

Fig. 115 Swing your legs back so that your hips leave the floor. Prop your hands against your hips.

Fig. 116 Slowly straighten up. When you have gone up as far as you can without strain, hold your position motionless for one to three minutes, as explained in the text which follows.

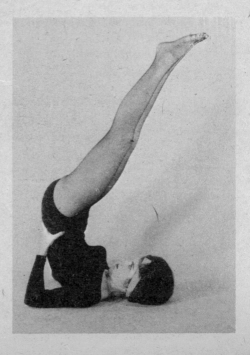

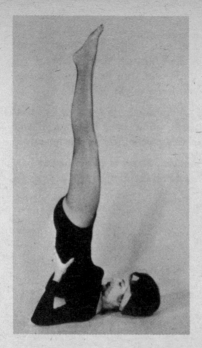

Fig. 117   The completed Shoulder Stand. The legs are now absolutely straight, and the body forms a right angle with the head. The chin presses against the chest. *The body is relaxed, not rigid.* The eyes may be closed.

Fig. 118   It is very important that you come out of the Shoulder Stand as instructed. The movements are similar to the Plough. Bend your knees and lower your legs as illustrated. Place the hands back on the floor.

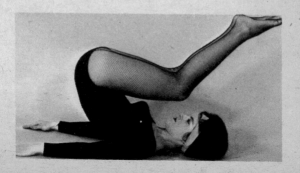

Fig. 119 Roll forward *slowly*, arching your neck backward to prevent your head from leaving the floor. Extend your legs straight upward.

Fig. 120 Very slowly, lower your legs to the floor. Once they touch, allow your body to go completely limp. Rest in this position for approximately thirty seconds.

The Shoulder Stand is performed only once and held from one to three minutes.

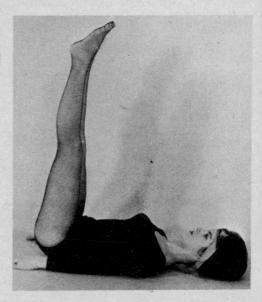

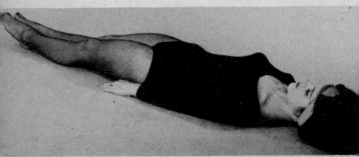

ACTION AND BENEFITS OF THE SHOULDER STAND

The Shoulder Stand has had a more pronounced effect in the improvement of blood circulation than any other single Yoga exercise. This will be obvious after you have performed the posture only a few times. You will feel the increased flow of blood into the thoracic, neck and head regions. The Shoulder Stand posture sends a rich supply of blood into the thyroid gland. The effects of this type of thyroid stimulation can be far-reaching, because the thyroid plays a most important role in many functions of the organism. Perhaps of greatest interest to the sedentary worker is the fact that the stimulation of the thyroid by means of the Shoulder Stand has helped an untold number of people to *control and redistribute weight!* This must certainly be a most encouraging feature of this exercise, especially when you can simultaneously feel a relaxation in the legs, as the pressure of the blood is relieved, and a lessening of weight on the organs and glands in the lower parts of the body. The exercise has proved helpful in certain disorders of the sexual organs. It has alleviated uterine difficulties, and prostate gland problems. *Practicing the Shoulder Stand for any of these disorders is contingent on the approval of one's physician.*

As was stated in connection with the Plough exercise, some individuals will have difficulty in raising the hips and waist from the floor; if so, the legs should be swung backward more quickly to gain the necessary momentum. The moment the hips leave the floor, brace your hands against them. If you positively cannot invert your body under its own power, then use the wall as an aid. Prop your legs against the wall and "walk up" the wall. Place a cushion beneath your head and shoulders. Remember that any angle of inversion is better than none. Once you have lifted your body into the position of *Fig. 115*, there need be no rush to attempt to straighten up. You may hold any position that is comfortable (or at least not strained) for thirty seconds to one minute in the beginning, then gradually increase the time. In almost all the exercises you can count the time periods for holding, but in the Shoulder and Head Stands you should have a timepiece where you can see it. Within a few days of practice most people are able to straighten up quite far, and the completed posture of *Fig. 117* should not be long in coming.

In *Fig. 117*, the completed posture, it is not necessary to keep the body rigid in military style. You may hold your legs limply in the air; if they or the feet feel as if they are "going to sleep," simply move them slowly to the sides or revolve the feet. You may even bend your knees slightly to help the circulation. All discomforts with respect to circulation usually disappear with practice. In coming out of the inverted position, follow the directions carefully so that you may perform the movements smoothly and gracefully and not break the continuity of the exercise. The point is to lower the legs and roll the trunk forward so that the head does not leave the floor.

Breathe slowly and deeply throughout all of the movements, especially while in the extreme position. This may prove difficult at first, but with a little practice the body will adjust itself to controlled breathing. Your eyes should be partially or fully closed. Attempt to take your mind off your immediate cares. You will feel wonderfully relaxed and refreshed when you have completed this posture and remained in a prone position for approximately thirty seconds to one minute.

HEAD STAND

Fig. 121 Sit on your heels; interlace your fingers as illustrated.

Fig. 122 Bend forward and rest your elbows, lower arms and hands to the floor, forming a triangle. Rest your toes on the floor.

Fig. 123 Lower your head to the floor so that the front of your head touches the floor and the back of your head rests against your locked fingers.

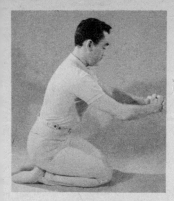

Fig. 121

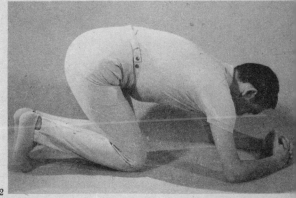

Fig. 122

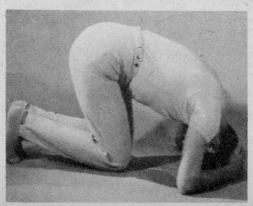

Fig. 123

Fig. 124 Place your full weight on your lower arms. Push up with your toes and raise your entire body as illustrated.

Fig. 125 Inch forward slowly with your toes until your knees are as close to your chest as possible. Bend your knees completely, push against the floor with your toes and attempt to bring the body into the position illustrated. This is the Modified Head Stand.

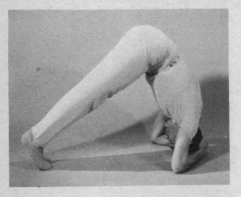

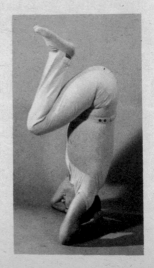

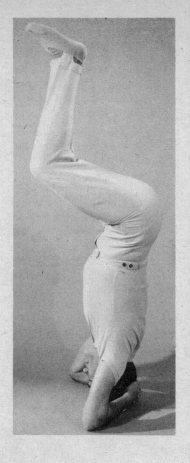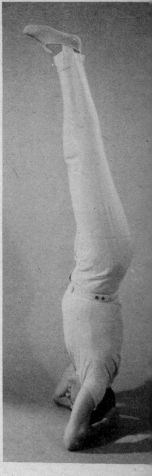

Fig. 126 To perform the Completed Head Stand, slowly straighten your knees and raise your legs into an intermediate position.

Fig. 127 The extreme posture.

Fig. 128 It is important to come out of the posture as directed. Bend your knees and slowly lower your legs.

Fig. 129 Lower the legs still farther, as illustrated. Keep your knees close in toward your chest.

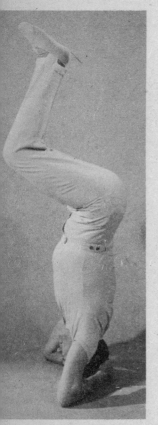
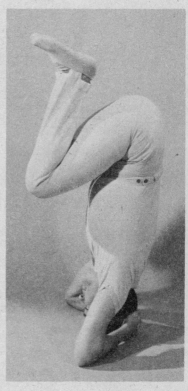

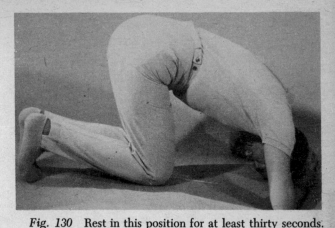

Fig. 130   Rest in this position for at least thirty seconds.

The Head Stand is performed only once and your extreme position is held from thirty seconds to three minutes.

ACTION AND BENEFITS OF THE HEAD STAND

Bringing the blood directly into the head benefits the sedentary worker greatly; nothing else can so quickly revitalize the brain. In addition to revitalizing the brain, the Head Stand has brought about improvement in vision, hearing and breathing. The sedentary worker will quickly recognize the Head Stand as one of his best friends and will understand how foolish are those who consider it a form of madness.

To stand on your head is not nearly as difficult as you may imagine. We do not do the head stand of the child or the acrobat; actually, by using the forearms we have a greater surface upon which to "stand" and support the weight of the body than is provided by the feet. There are two parts to the Head Stand, and we perfect the first part or Modified position of *Fig. 125* before going on to the Completed posture of *Fig. 127*. We attempt in this posture, as in all of the Yoga techniques, to obtain complete control at every point of the exercise. This control will enable one to perform all of the postures, including the Head Stand, in a slow-motion pace, thus deriving the most possible benefit.

Figures 121-24 should not offer any difficulty. The secret of success with the Head Stand lies in the correct execution of the movements in *Fig. 125*. In inching forward, you must keep your back in the position illustrated and *bring the bent knees in toward your chest as far as possible*. This concentrates all the weight of your body in a relatively small area so that the balance may be shifted when the legs spring lightly into the air. The Modified position is as far as you should go at first. Do not try to straighten your legs until you have completely mastered this posture. When you are ready to attempt the Completed Head Stand, continue from the position of *Fig. 125* by raising your legs very slowly one inch at a time. If you try to spring into the vertical posture all at once, you will never master the Head Stand. Whatever extreme position you choose to maintain should be held for thirty seconds in the beginning and gradually increased to approximately two to three minutes. If thirty seconds seems too long, you may begin with fifteen or even ten seconds. Conversely, once you are secure in the posture you may wish to hold it five minutes or longer. Maximum time for advanced students should be ten minutes.

If you are skpetical about being able to maintain your balance in the Head Stand, use the wall for support. Place yourself about one foot from the wall and let your feet rest against the wall as you roll forward in *Fig. 125*. If you do use the wall, continue to push yourself easily away from it with your feet and attempt to balance yourself. You should use a small pillow under your head to prevent any soreness and also surround yourself with a few pillows and blankets so that if you lose your balance you will be protected. In the first few attempts you may feel dizzy or somewhat uncomfortable, but after about a week of practice this feeling almost always disappears and never returns. It is most important that in coming out of the posture you do not drop the body with a jolt or bang your feet against the floor. Lower your body slowly, maintaining complete control. You can accomplish this by carefully learning the movements of *Figs. 128-29*. Always rest with your head on the floor, as indicated in *Fig. 130*. Never jump up immediately, because the sudden change can make you dizzy. *Persons with high blood pressure, cardiac conditions or a history of head injury should consult their physicians before attempting the Head Stand.*

The Head Stand is the last in our series of five postures for improvement of the blood circulation. Not all of these techniques will be performed the same day. We will be performing the Complete Breath *each day* and rotating the other four exercises over a period of four days.

Muscle Tone

and Firmness

The problem here is obvious: The sedentary worker does not exert sufficient muscular effort to retain the resilience of the muscles. All muscles must receive stress to remain in condition, and in the case of almost every sedentary worker this does not occur. He is certain, therefore, to lose muscle tone through the years. The problem of maintaining muscle tone is complicated by a fact that has been mentioned previously: The average worker associates muscular fitness with *heavy* muscular work requiring a great deal of effort. He is not inclined to engage in such work or exercise and generally ends up doing no real muscular exercise at all. The muscles gradually deteriorate; the resulting flabbiness and general fatigue are well known to sedentary workers.

The Yoga strengthening and developing exercises that follow require a minimum of effort and time for a maximum return in firming. Also, *all* of the body's muscles are involved in a few movements, and the exercises have been designed in such a way that anyone, regardless of how weakened he has become, can rebuild and develop *progressively*. There is as much challenge in each of these Yoga techniques as one wishes to accept. Not only will you find yourself exercising muscles of which you are well aware (arm, leg and abdominal muscles) but you will also bring into play vital muscles of the groin, back and neck, of whose loss of resilience you may be unaware.

Only four exercises are in the following series, but they are extremely dynamic and produce quick results. If you follow the instructions you will never become sore or experience the next-day discomfort of muscles strained or overworked by strenuous exercise or sports. Firm muscles preserve the good appearance and feeling of the body; muscles in the process of atrophying make the body appear old long before its time. There is no reason why the sedentary worker should not maintain good muscle tone throughout his life.

SIDE RAISE

Fig. 131 Lie on your left side in the position illustrated. The legs are together. Your left hand rests firmly against your cheek.

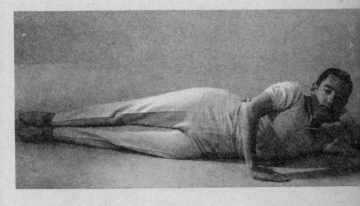

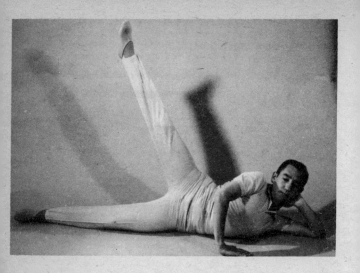

Fig. 132 Slowly raise your right leg as high as you can. Hold for a count of 5; lower slowly.

Fig. 133 Push down hard with your right hand and raise both legs as illustrated. The legs come up directly from the side without swaying off to the right or left. Keep your legs together. Hold for a count of 5. Slowly lower the legs and repeat.

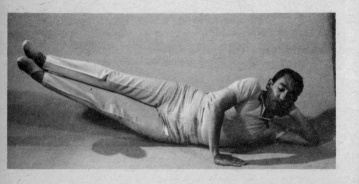

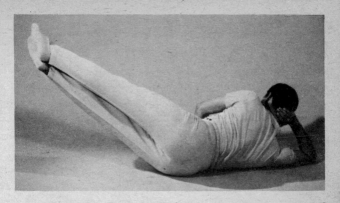

Fig. 134 Perform the identical movements on your right side. First raise only the left leg once, then both legs.

Perform the Side Raise as follows: once with the right leg and twice with both legs; once with the left leg and twice with both legs. Hold each extreme position for a count of 5.

ACTION AND BENEFITS OF THE SIDE RAISE

The Side Raise is a toning and firming movement for the legs, thighs, hips and buttocks. The arm will also become firm through the pushing-down movements. The position of *Fig. 132* is relatively easy, but effective for the inside of the thigh and the groin. Remember to raise and lower the leg slowly. *Figure 133* is not easy and requires effort. This effort is most effective for streamlining (especially hips, waist and buttocks). You have to push down hard with your hand and bring the legs up *together* with the feet touching. You will lose the firming properties if the legs are not held together. It is also most important that you attempt to bring the legs up *directly from the side* rather than allow them to move forward or backward. In the beginning the legs may only raise a few inches from the floor, but as the necessary muscle tone is developed they will go increasingly higher. You may also find that you do better on one side than the other. This simply indicates that there is more muscle tone on the stronger side.

BACK PUSH-UP

Fig. 135 Place body in position illustrated. Heels are in as far as possible.

Fig. 136 Push down with your hands and feet and raise the body a moderate distance from the floor. Hold for a count of 10.

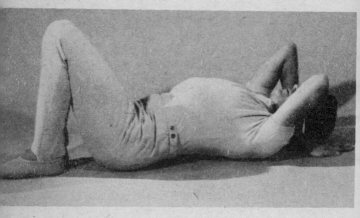

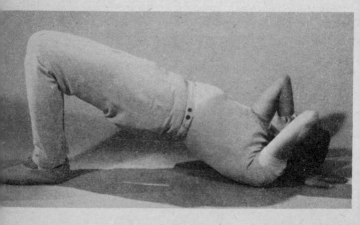

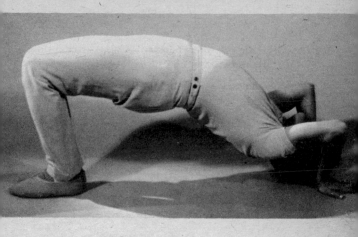

Fig. 137 Arch the neck so that the top of the head rests on the floor; raise the body as far as possible. Hold for a count of 10. Slowly lower the body and repeat.

Perform the Back Push-Up three times: once as in *Fig. 136* and twice as in *Fig. 137*.

ACTION AND BENEFITS OF THE BACK PUSH-UP

This firming exercise is self-explanatory. A few pointers should be of aid. In *Fig. 135*, either the hands may rest on the floor (as illustrated) or the exercise can be performed on the fingertips to strengthen the fingers. The position of *Fig. 136* is assumed to "warm up." The extreme position of *Fig. 137* has the neck arched and the top of the head on the floor so that the body may be raised considerably higher than in *Fig. 136*. (An even more advanced position can be attained with practice.) Attempt to keep your knees together when lifting the body. This is effective for the legs and buttocks. Push down hard with your hands or fingers to help to strengthen your hands, wrists and upper arms. You will also find the neck strengthened by the arching movement of *Fig. 137*.

LOCUST

Fig. 138 Lie on your abdomen. Rest your chin on the floor. Make two fists and place them near your sides.

Fig. 139 Push down with your fists and slowly raise your right leg as high as possible. Hold for a count of 5. Lower the right leg and perform the same movement with the left leg.

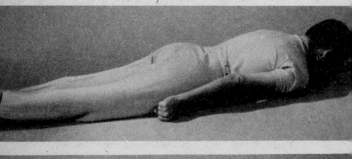

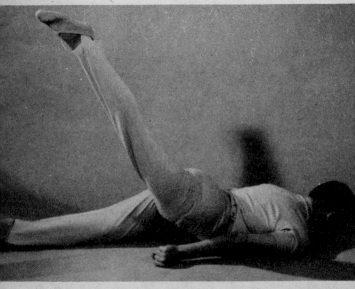

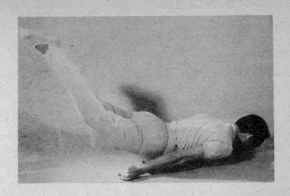

Fig. 140 Inhale and hold your breath. Push down very hard with your fists and attempt to raise both legs from the floor. *Keep your chin on the floor* and the knees as straight as possible. Hold whatever extreme position you can attain for a count of 5. Lower your legs slowly with control, rest a moment and repeat.

Fig. 141 A more advanced position in which both the legs and the groin area are lifted from the floor. The knees are bent in this extreme posture. The position is held for a count of 5.

Perform the Locust once with each leg and twice with both legs.

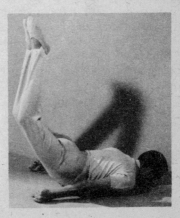

ACTION AND BENEFITS OF THE LOCUST

The Locust is the perfect exercise, especially for sedentary workers, for regaining muscle tone and strength in the areas of the upper legs and groin.

In *Fig. 138*, place the hands with the *thumbs down* on the floor. Keep the arms close to your sides. Place the head so that the mouth, rather than the point of the chin, rests on the floor. *Figure 139* should present no problem. It is a fine loosening movement. In *Fig. 140*, it is completely natural to be able to raise the legs only a few inches from the floor during initial attempts. You must first inhale and hold the breath, because this builds stamina for the lifting. Also, the fists must push down very hard against the floor (an excellent movement for firming and strengthening the entire arm). For added effectiveness try to keep the legs close together and do not bend the knees. After the count of 5, lower your legs slowly (don't collapse); exhale as you come down. When you have done the exercise twice, rest your cheek on the floor and allow your body to relax completely.

In addition to the obvious firming and strengthening properties of the Locust, these movements, according to the Yogis, stimulate the organs and glands of the groin and abdomen. This is particularly true of the advanced posture of *Fig. 141*. Here you can see that the body resembles the grasshopper or locust. Sufficient strength and control have now been gained to lift the groin from the floor and, for this reason, the knees are bent. This position may seem far beyond your ability at present, but repetitions will develop the weakened muscles involved.

LIE DOWN-SIT UP

Fig. 142 Sit as illustrated.

Fig. 143 In very slow motion, without the aid of your hands, lower your trunk toward the floor.

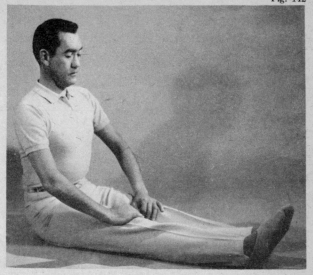

Fig. 142

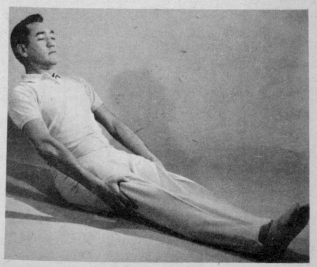

Fig. 143

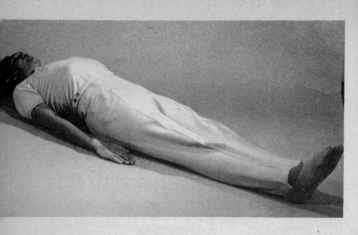

Fig. 144 Continue the movement until your back rests on the floor.

Fig. 145 Without pause, bend your knees and bring them in toward the abdomen. Next, straighten your legs as illustrated. Then, in very slow motion, lower your legs to the floor.

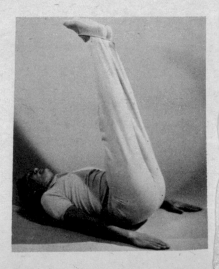

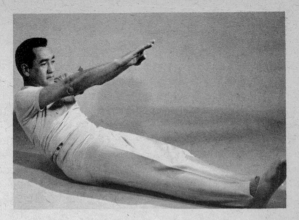

Fig. 146 Without pause, and in very slow motion, begin to raise your trunk as illustrated. Try not to use your hands.

Fig. 147 When reaching the sitting position, slowly slide your hands as far as possible down your legs. Without pause, slowly straighten up into the original sitting position and repeat.

Perform the entire routine twice.

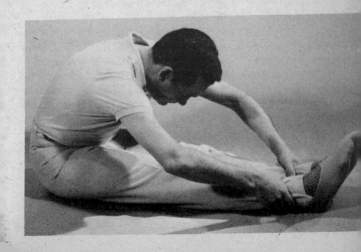

ACTION AND BENEFITS OF THE LIE DOWN-SIT UP

A great deal of firming is involved in this exercise, which is concentrated in the abdominal area. If you practice the movements of these exercises as directed, you will streamline your body through the hips and waist and find that the entire abdominal area becomes firm and solid.

This series of movements is performed in continuous motion; there are no holding positions. You will notice the continual use of the word *slowly*. Strictly observe this direction in your practice, not only for this exercise but as it appears throughout all of the Yoga postures. If you are used to doing the calisthenic-type exercises with their quick 1-2, 1-2-3-4 movements you will have to continually remind yourself of the slow motion in Yoga. Once this slowness has been impressed upon the body you will find it infinitely more natural and meaningful than the quick movements.

In *Fig. 143* you will feel the muscle toning that takes place as you attempt to lower your trunk slowly as instructed. If you find this movement too difficult, you can use your elbows to help. The movements of *Fig. 145* are the same as those used in the Plough and the Shoulder Stand, in which the bent knees are straightened into the air and lowered very slowly for abdominal firming. The sitting-up movement of *Fig. 146* is the most difficult part of the exercise, and many will find that they must use their elbows to help push up until the abdominal muscles have been sufficiently strengthened. Often a quick thrust of the trunk from the lying position will be helpful in the first attempt to raise the trunk. Try to keep the legs on the floor throughout the lifting of the trunk. The movements of *Fig. 147* provide an additional stretch for the legs and back and add symmetry and balance to the entire exercise.

Balance – Grace – Poise

These are important qualities of the body that the sedentary worker may not even consider, much less practice to maintain. Nor are they to be considered as solely feminine attributes, since balance and poise imply good co-ordination and timing. The physical organism is an instrument of incredible beauty, and one who is aware of this shows it in all of his movements—even in the most minor gesture of head or hand. Such a person always has a presence and a beauty which, although often intangible, is very real; it is felt by all who come in contact with him.

The sedentary worker, however, confined largely to his desk five days a week, growing stiff, weak, flabby and experiencing numerous tensions and frustrations, may easily lose sight of the fact that his physical as well as mental condition can undergo a remarkable positive change when he becomes aware of this beauty within and the fact that he can begin to exert real control over his body if he wishes. All of the Yoga postures are designed to provide such control in one form or another. Certain exercises emphasize balance. We have already performed several of these: the Toe Twist, Rishi's Posture, the Shoulder Stand and the Head Stand are examples. The Arm and Leg Stretch that follows is the most intensive movement to impart balance and co-ordination.

ARM AND LEG STRETCH

Fig. 148   In a standing position slowly raise your right arm straight overhead.

Fig. 149   Slowly raise your left leg behind you and hold the left foot with your left hand. The right arm can come forward to help the balance.

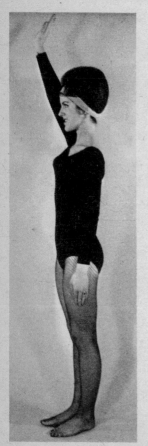
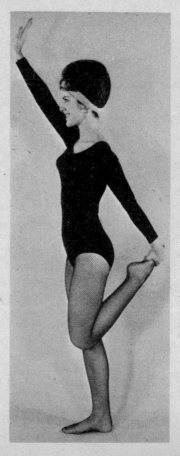

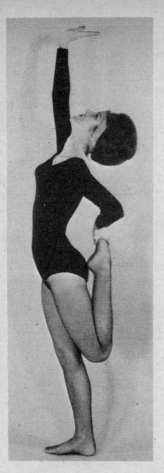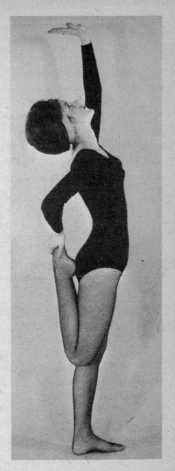

Fig. 150 Slowly bring your right arm back and your left foot up as far as possible without strain. Drop your head back. Hold without motion for a count of 5. Bring the arm and leg down.

Fig. 151 Perform the identical movements on the opposite side.

Perform the Arm and Leg Stretch twice on each side, alternating the sides.

ACTION AND BENEFITS OF THE ARM AND LEG STRETCH

The Arm and Leg Stretch is not only a control and balance exercise but a powerful movement for the spine and thighs. In *Fig. 149*, stand easily, not rigidly, on the right foot. This will make balancing easier. *Figure 150* shows the completed posture and the stretch. Note that the arm is upraised and the elbow is not bent; the foot is held firmly and pulled up as far as possible without strain; the head is dropped back and the eyes look up. The posture is one of great form and symmetry. You are almost certain to lose your balance in the beginning. As in the Toe Twist, you must never laugh at yourself or become discouraged. When you begin to totter, don't hop about on one foot attempting to regain control. Drop the arm and leg as gracefully as possible, pause a moment and begin again. In the beginning it may take three or four attempts to complete one stretch, but there is no other way of learning control except through repetition.

If you find it absolutely impossible to maintain your balance after repeated attempts, then you can rest your right side against the wall when attempting the position of *Fig. 148*, and the left side against the wall when attempting the position of *Fig. 151*. As you become more secure and accomplished, you will find that an even more advanced position (*Fig. 150*) is made possible by bringing the arm farther back and placing the foot in the small of the back. Always proceed slowly. This is a powerful stretch.

Internal Exercising

With the concept of "internal exercising" one can begin to truly appreciate the profundity of Yoga. In almost all systems of exercise the emphasis is placed on the muscles, with the heart and lungs occasionally mentioned. In Yoga, the muscular system is not considered more important than the respiratory, circulatory or endocrine systems. Hence we have used the term *internal exercising* to indicate that the organs and glands throughout the entire organism will be methodically stimulated. Let us see how some of this is accomplished: There is no exercise which can be of more help to the brain, eyes, ears and nose than the Head Stand. The pituitary gland is also involved in the Head Stand. The thyroid gland is intensively stimulated by the Shoulder Stand. The heart is involved in the Head and Shoulder Stands and the Locust, as are the reproductive organs and glands. The kidneys are stimulated by means of the Cobra and Bow. Numerous other examples can be cited.

The sedentary worker should realize that the Yoga postures offer a type of internal stimulation not provided by his usual activities or even his hobbies or sports. This should be an added incentive to practice Yoga.

Perhaps the Abdominal Lift is the most obvious of all the Yoga exercises in which internal stimulation is involved. Here one feels immediately the benefits which must result from the practice of this technique. Imagine being able to stimulate the stomach, colon, intestines, liver, kidneys, gall bladder, pancreas, reproductive organs—all with one movement! These are the properties of the Abdominal Lift; for the sedentary worker such an exercise is invaluable. Indeed, it is a serious error to think that we can have a successful National Physical Fitness program without this type of internal exercising. Note carefully what you experience with the Abdominal Lift. It will be most revealing.

ABDOMINAL LIFT

Fig. 152 From a standing position, place your body in the posture illustrated. Note very carefully the position of the feet. The knees are slightly bent; the hands rest on the upper thighs with all fingers turned inward. Allow the abdomen to relax.

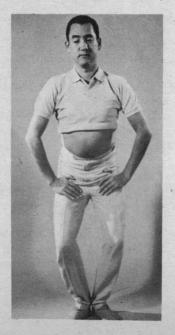

Fig. 153 Study *Figs. 153* and *154*. It is important to realize that the lifting of the abdomen as illustrated can be successfully accomplished only if all air is completely exhaled from your lungs and no air is allowed to enter while the abdominal movements are being performed.

Therefore, exhale fully and attempt to lift the abdomen as indicated. Make certain no air is allowed to enter your lungs during the lift. Hold the lift for one second.

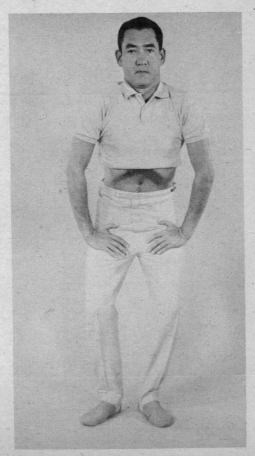

Fig. 154 A close-up of the lift.

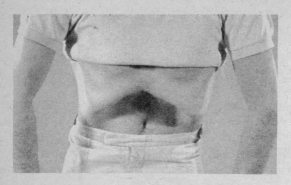

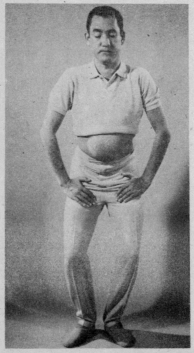

Fig. 155

Fig. 155 After the one-second hold, push out very forcibly with the abdominal muscles and attempt to "snap" the entire abdomen out as far as possible. Repeat the movement.

Perform as many movements as possible without inhaling. This may be three, five and gradually ten and more to each exhalation. Then stand up straight and rest a few moments. Go back into the squatting position and repeat five times.

ACTION AND BENEFITS OF THE ABDOMINAL LIFT

The Abdominal Lift is the very finest natural movement you can perform to stimulate and promote the functioning of the visceral organs and glands. It helps to promote peristaltic action, relieving and preventing constipation. It reduces flabbiness in the waist and maintains the resilience of the abdominal muscles, thus helping to prevent the abdomen from dropping.

Success in this exercise is a matter of practice, and one must not become discouraged if he cannot perform the lift completely during the first few days. The technique may seem peculiar until you catch on to the knack of doing the movements *while the breath is exhaled.* All of the air must be exhaled and kept out in order to create a vacuum, or you will not be able to lift sufficiently to form the large, necessary "hollow." If in the beginning, however, you are able to only *contract* the abdomen you are already benefiting from this movement. But remember that the eventual goal is not only to contract the abdomen but to *raise* it.

When attempting the lift in *Figs. 153* and *154,* push down hard on your thighs; do not allow yourself to lean over farther than you see in the illustration. Do the movements forcefully and rhythmically, even if you can do only one or two movements to each exhalation. The steady rhythm, not the speed, is important. This is one of the very few quick-motion Yoga techniques. In *Fig. 155* the abdomen is not allowed merely to fall back to its normal position; it is "shot" or "snapped" out in a vigorous, forceful movement by the abdominal muscles. When you stand up to rest after each group of lifts, try not to fidget or grow restless. Stand quietly and breathe deeply for a few moments until you are rested, then repeat. Within a few weeks of practice you should be able to do forty to fifty lifts within the five repetitions. This exercise must always be done when the stomach is empty.

Part Two

Yoga

During the Workday

It is gratifying to note that more and more companies are realizing the value of brief exercise periods during working hours. It would seem obvious that the efficiency of the worker will increase if he has the opportunity either to avoid or to relieve the onset of deadly physical and emotional fatigue that occurs with astonishing regularity during predictable morning and afternoon hours. Having become aware of this, some large manufacturing plants now have facilities for workers to enjoy an exercise break as they do a coffee break. Unfortunately, the number of enlightened companies in this regard is still quite limited, and most sedentary workers must rely on their own ingenuity for a practical exercise break. With the four Yoga exercises that follow, anyone can have this break within a matter of five minutes and feel wonderfully refreshed! The first is a standing technique that offers a general stretching of all of the major muscles and ligaments where tension accumulates. The next three are sitting exercises: one for the spine; the second, the neck; and the third, the lungs.

Noteworthy in this series is the fact that, like all of the Yoga techniques, it considers emotional and mental aspects of the organism as well as the physical. This becomes tremendously important when one realizes the innumerable forces which must be coped with during the workday. The average office is, psychologically speaking, a most complex structure, where the conflicts of interests and personalities are often overwhelming. Frustrations and hostilities (as well as the physical discomforts already discussed), that are bound to arise in some degree within every worker, take their toll on the organism. It is probably unnecessary to elaborate on this point; it is known only too well. To imply that the practice of Yoga can eliminate such negative conditions may be overly optimistic. But it is highly realistic to state that they can certainly be reduced by the Yoga techniques, both in the office and at home. In addition, the worker receives a great psychological boost when he realizes the dynamic weapon that Yoga provides—one that he can use whenever necessary.

Take the five minutes required to perform the following group of office exercises. Do them twice a day—at midmorning and midafternoon. Within one week you will be fully convinced of their value. It is good to have privacy if possible. If not, do them at your desk or anywhere that is convenient. Your fellow workers will very quickly become curious and probably want to learn the movements.

In addition to four suggested exercises (descriptions follow), three other exercises that we have already learned can be added to the routine. They are the Leg Clasp, the Elbow Exercise and the Eye Exercise.

CHEST EXPANSION

Fig. 156 In a standing position, gracefully raise your arms and bring your hands into the posture illustrated.

Fig. 157 Slowly stretch your arms straight out before you. Feel the elbows stretch.

Fig. 158 Bring your arms straight back as far as possible, in line with your shoulders. When you can go no farther, drop your arms so that you can clasp your hands and interlock your fingers. Keep your trunk erect. Do not bend forward.

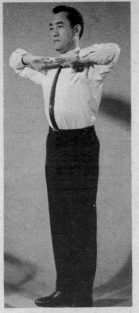

Fig. 156

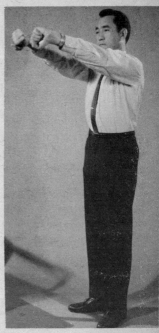

Fig. 157

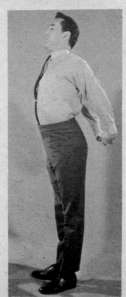

Fig. 158

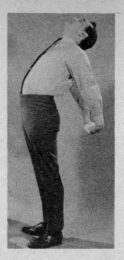

Fig. 159 Keep your arms raised as high as possible and bend backward very slowly. Do not bend your knees. When you have bent backward a moderate distance, hold for a count of 5.

Fig. 160 Now bring your arms up and over your back as you slowly bend forward. Keep your arms and legs straight.

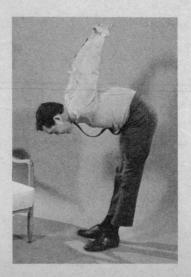

Fig. 161 Continue to bend forward as far as possible without strain. Hold for a count of 10.

Fig. 162 Straighten up slightly so that you can extend your right leg out to the side. Then bend forward as before, but now aim your forehead toward your right knee. (This is to stretch away tensions which accumulate in the knee and thigh.) Hold for a count of 10. The left knee may bend to aid in the stretch.

Fig. 163 Perform the identical movements with the left leg, as illustrated. Hold for a count of 10. When you have completed the movements, straighten up very slowly and repeat.

Perform the entire routine of the Chest Expansion twice.

Fig. 161

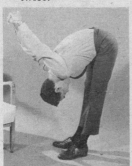

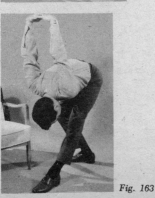

Fig. 162

Fig. 163

SIMPLE TWIST

Fig. 164   Cross the right leg over the left.

Fig. 165   Grip the seat of the chair with your right hand. Cross your left arm over your right knee and hold your left knee as illustrated.

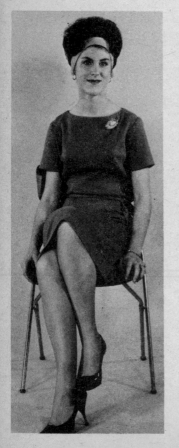
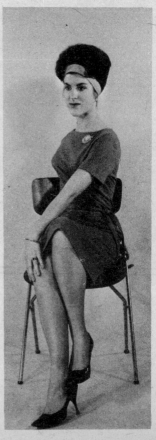

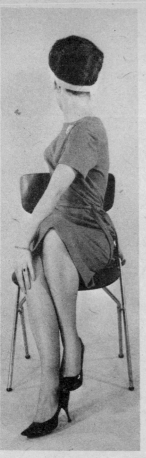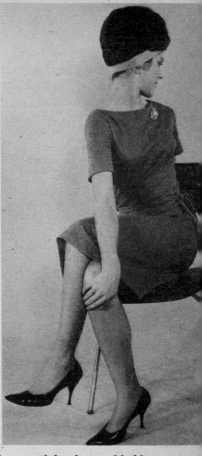

Fig. 166 Gripping the seat of the chair and holding your left knee firmly, slowly twist as far as possible to your right. Hold for a count of 5. Turn forward and relax a moment. Then repeat.

Fig. 167 Perform the identical movements on the opposite side.

Perform the Simple Twist twice on each side.

NECK ROLL

Fig. 168 Slowly bend your head forward and allow your chin to rest against your chest. Hold for a count of 5. Close your eyes.

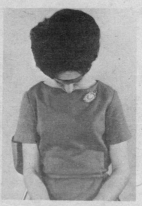

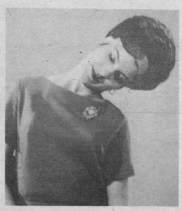

Fig. 169 Slowly roll and twist your head to the extreme left. Hold for 5.

Fig. 170 Slowly roll and twist your head to the extreme backward position. Feel your chin and throat muscles stretching. Hold for 5.

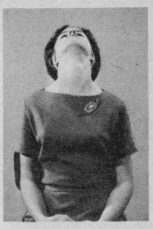

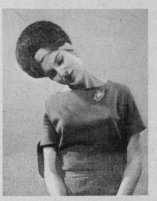

Fig. 171 Slowly roll and twist your head to the extreme right. Hold for 5.

Perform the routine three times. If more loosening is needed, perform as many times as necessary.

CHARGING BREATH

Fig. 172 Sit as illustrated. The first movement of the Charging Breath is identical with that which we learned in the Complete Breath. As you inhale, push out with your abdominal muscles so that the abdomen is distended as far as possible.

Fig. 173 Now with a sudden, forceful movement, pull in and contract your abdomen. If you do this forcefully, the air will be literally "shot" from your lungs and pass out through the nose. (The mouth is closed.) It is difficult to depict this movement in the illustration, but with this forceful contraction you allow the air to make a strong hissing sound as it is forced through the lungs and nostrils. If you perform this movement strongly enough you should be able to feel a shaking of the entire chest area.

This is a continuous inhalation and exhalation. You do not pause between the movements. Perform fifteen of these movements.

Fig. 174 When you have completed the series of fifteen movements, slowly take a Complete Breath. Retain the air in your lungs and bring the middle finger of your right hand into the position illustrated.

Fig. 175 Retain the breath and vigorously tap the entire chest area with the finger. Start at the highest part of the chest—in the clavicle area—and tap across and down into the lowest part of the rib cage. Put your hand down and slowly exhale.

Perform the entire routine of the Charging Breath, that is, the fifteen charging movements, the Complete Breath and the tapping, five times.

Fig. 172

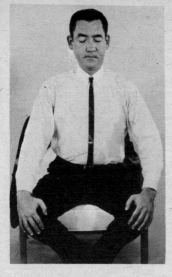

Fig. 173

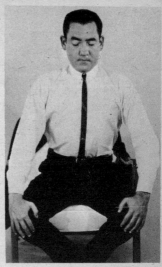

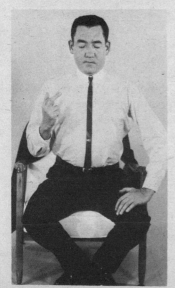

Fig. 174

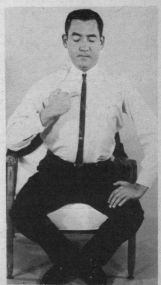

Fig. 175

ACTION AND BENEFITS OF THE CHARGING BREATH

This is a highly invigorating as well as cleansing technique. You must practice this exercise in a definite rhythm with the inhalations and exhalations equal in time. You can begin as slowly as you wish and gradually increase the tempo. If you attempt to go too quickly in the beginning, you will run out of air. The abdomen is pushed *out* as the air is taken *in*. (This, in a sense, is like loading a gun with a bullet. Here, the lungs are loaded with air.) In the second part of the exercise, the air is "shot" out of the lungs by pulling the trigger (the quick contraction of the abdomen). Careful attention, therefore, must be given to how the air is taken in and how it is expelled. The relatively quick inhalation and exhalation charges the organism with the life-force (*prana*) in the air. The tapping of the chest is for lung cell stimulation. Tap vigorously and throughout the entire chest as directed. The movement is similar to the way a physician taps the chest during an examination—a rhythmic, hammer-like action.

You may find yourself coughing during or after this exercise. This is natural and beneficial if you are a heavy smoker or if there is excessive mucus in your lungs or sinus cavities. This Charging Breath also acts in a cleansing manner helping to loosen congestion. The Yogi therefore considers this as a hygienic practice.

It is interesting to note that this exercise heats the body if performed fifteen or twenty times. In a cold climate the Yogi often uses the technique for heating purposes.

Part Three

Special Problems

Through the centuries it has been observed that as a by-product of the practice of physical Yoga, many discomforts and illnesses, some major, some minor, have been affected in a very positive manner. Whether or not specific exercises and postures were originally designed for certain afflictions is difficult to determine because of the antiquity of these exercises, but there is no question of their genuine therapeutic value. The Yogic claims in the original Sanskrit texts and those currently made by the various Hatha Yoga institutes in India and other parts of the world are very authoritative with regard to the healing properties of Yoga. People attending such institutions often study physical Yoga for the express purpose of attempting to cure major diseases, and these efforts have proven highly successful, as the author well knows.

In this book we shall make no such claims regarding the use of Yoga for treatment of diseases. The exercises are never to be used as a substitute for competent medical advice and therapy. But there are many minor discomforts and problems to which the Yoga techniques may well be applied, once the consent of one's physician has been obtained. Most physicians who have seen the Yoga exercises performed have offered their complete approval, because the mildness of the techniques makes them particularly advantageous for those who must exercise with caution and those who wish to remain physically fit but can afford no possibility of strain.*

Seven problems prevalent among sedentary workers will be discussed in the following pages. Specifically, these are: weight control, posture, headaches and tension, constipation, exceptional stiffness, insomnia and poor breathing. For each we will offer simple but very effective exercises. When dealing with a particular problem you may find it advantageous to perform the given exercises more than the suggested number of repetitions and to practice them more than once daily. You must always remember that the problems discussed here (as well as many others) have usually taken some years to become manifest, and it is therefore unrealistic to expect some type of magical cure within a few days of practice. The peoples of the western world have been conditioned to hope for instant, "miracle" cures for their afflictions. But if the laws of nature have been abused for prolonged periods, no sudden reversal of the resultant condition can be expected. The Yoga postures rebuild and strengthen—a process that obviously requires time. Of course, each physical organism is different and responds accordingly. You will probably find that you notice relatively quick progress with the problems of headaches and tension, constipation and insomnia. But weight control, posture, exceptional stiffness and poor breathing will take longer to rectify.

Nature is *with* you when you practice Yoga because your body wants and needs the exact type of stretching and stimulation which these techniques provide. Persevere, and you can look forward to wonderful, natural results.

---

* A film titled *Use of Yoga Exercises in Physical Medicine,* prepared by the author in collaboration with O. L. Huddleston, M.D. of the California Rehabilitation Center, Santa Monica, California was presented before the American Congress of Physical Medicine and Rehabilitation at its 40th Annual Session (New York City, 1962).

Weight Control

The relative inactivity of the sedentary worker contributes to the problem of excess weight. As a group, sedentary workers are more prone to excess weight than are employees in any other classification. Yoga offers a unique and fascinating approach to the problem of excess weight. First, it is essential to understand that the weight control problem cannot be treated en masse. That is, as far as we are concerned, each sedentary worker who is overweight has an *individual* problem because his metabolism and certain other vital factors are necessarily different from those of his fellow workers. Because of these differences, the amount of food that constitutes overeating and the amount of activity that constitutes sufficient exercise vary with the individual. In your office you can see many workers who eat heavily at mealtime, pack in several between-meal snacks and barely move out of their chairs during the workday, yet are far less overweight than those who may be watching their diets and are very active during working hours! What accounts for this apparent discrepancy? The fact is: Their bodies function differently.

Thus it follows that it is of the utmost importance for each person to make every effort to "Know thyself," that is, to know what *your* correct weight should be (at what weight *you* know you are functioning at your best), exactly how the foods that you are eating affect *you* and the value various sports and exercise routines have for *you*. This implies complete self-reliance. It entails turning away from the charts on the scales or those listed in the Sunday supplements (as though millions of people had the identical skeleton and bone structure) and making a self-examination. If you are large-boned your weight and measurements must be different than those of one who is small-boned. If a large-boned woman attempts to model her measurements after the mannequins of the fashion magazines she will not only be unsuccessful but she can actually find herself in serious physical trouble. From the Yogic viewpoint it is not only unnatural but often harmful and even dangerous to attempt to reduce excess weight through the "hi-protein" fad, which greatly increases the metabolic activity. The same can be true for the steam bath, the "miracle" 21-day diet, the substitution of pills, powders, wafers and liquids for the nourishment of food, the push-and-pull gadgets and the quick, forceful, strenuous movements of calisthenics. What is more, excess weight taken off in this manner will return in almost every case when the program is discontinued. Why? Because the above procedures are unnatural; they do not assist nature's plan, but *oppose* it!

It is the concept of Yoga that the wisdom and intelligence of your body are much greater than all of the magazine "miracle" diets, the ingenious exercising machines, the calorie counting charts and so on. Do you know that you have this great wisdom within your own organism? Most people have allowed this power to fall asleep. It is our objective, with all of the Yoga techniques you will learn and practice, to stimulate and reawaken this life-force so that it can help you do all of the things you would like to do. When the life-force becomes active and dynamic we can begin to feel very acutely those things which are of benefit to our organism and those which are of harm. We know with a powerful instinct which foods to avoid, the amount of sleep we individually require, and in all aspects of life we become, with a great conviction of being right, our own guides. This concept of looking more and more to ourselves for guidance in all phases of living is a fundamental objective of the science of Yoga. Extraordinarily enough, this objective is attained to a great extent through the physical postures!

It is natural to want to have a diet and an exercise plan to follow when one desires to lose weight. In my book, *Be Young with Yoga*, the student is provided with certain *principles* of nutrition instead of hard and fast rules regarding the counting of calories, the intake of protein and so forth. This enables the student to experiment with these principles (which seem to conform to nature's plan) and their reaction on his individual organism. In this way, each may eventually determine for himself his own path. If you will make a sincere effort to find out what foods are best for you, your organism will aid you in every possible way. You do not have to fight your body; you simply have to harmonize with it and listen to what it is asking of you. Is this not a most intelligent method?

Now as to the exercise routine: All of the Yoga exercises in this book are going to help you control and normalize your weight. The special routine of techniques in the following pages are to be practiced specifically for stimulating the thyroid and firming and strengthening certain areas of the body. You will find that when these usually flabby areas are firmed, weight can be much more easily removed, as well as correctly proportioned. Regardless of your structure, as your muscles and skin become taut and firm, your posture and carriage erect and your movements graceful and poised, you will cease to appear overweight or underweight. The beauty of your own body, as you define your structure, will be a revelation! You will appear confident, vital and in harmony with nature—and this will be especially true when you radiate the internal health and optimism which results from "getting with yourself."

Finally, any serious weight problem should always be dealt with by your physician and you should consult him before undertaking a special program of diet and exercise. It is also important to point out that many of the Yoga relaxing exercises, particularly the breathing and stretching techniques should help to diminish the unnatural desire of the compulsive eater. This desire is often due to nervous disturbances, and if the nervousness can be alleviated, the desire often disappears. Underweight people often find that when they are able to relax, their assimilation is much improved and their body weight becomes normal.

ROLL TWIST

Fig. 176 Stand erect with your feet together and your hands on your hips. Bend forward slightly as illustrated.

Fig. 177 *Slowly roll and twist in a small circle* to your left. Keep your knees straight and do not move your legs. Only the trunk rolls and twists. Hold the position without movement for a count of 2.

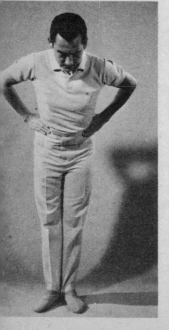
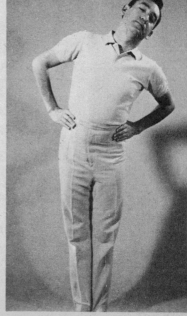

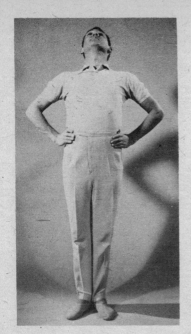

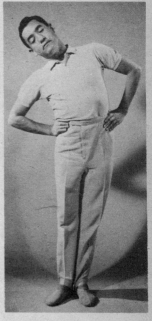

Fig. 178 Slowly roll and twist your trunk in a small circle to the backward position. Hold for a count of 2.

Fig. 179 Slowly roll and twist in a small circle to your right. Hold for a count of 2.

Fig. 180 Slowly roll and twist in a small circle to the original position. Hold for a count of 2. Now bend forward several inches farther than when you began. Compare *Figs. 176* and *180*.

Fig. 181 The object is to now make a wider circle with your trunk. Slowly roll and twist in a wider circle to your left. Compare *Figs. 177* and *181*.

Continue the wider circle with the trunk by rolling and twisting first to the backward position and then to the right. Hold each position for a count of 2. Then return to the forward position of *Fig. 180*.

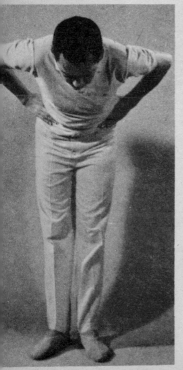

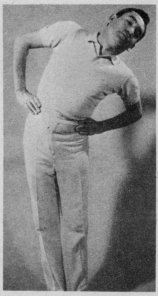

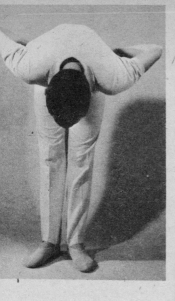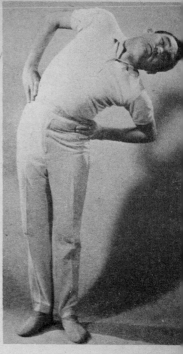

Fig. 182 The object now is to make the widest circle possible without strain. Bend forward as far as possible.

Fig. 183 Roll and twist as far as possible to your left. Compare with *Fig. 181*. Continue the widest circle possible by rolling and twisting to the backward, right and forward positions. Hold each for a rhythmic count of 2. When you have completed the movements, straighten up and rest a few moments. Then repeat the identical movements from each of the three positions.

Perform the Roll Twist five times. If you are attempting to reduce in the waist and hips, perform ten times. Do the movements rhythmically, pausing in each position for a count of 2. Keep the image of making the widening circles as you roll and twist your trunk.

HIP BEND

Fig. 184 Stand erect with your feet together. Raise your arms overhead so that they are parallel with palms facing each other.

Fig. 185 *Slowly* bend to your left side from the waist. Keep your knees straight and make sure your arms remain parallel. Hold without motion for a count of 5.

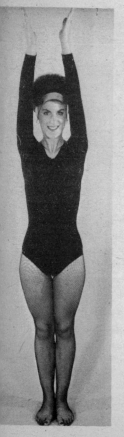
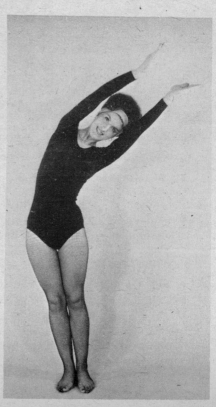

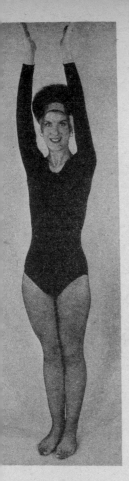

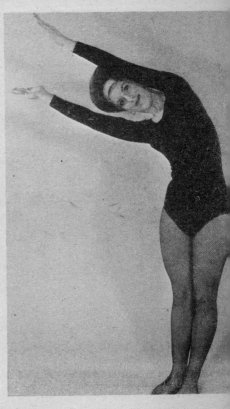

Fig. 186 Slowly straighten up.

Fig. 187 Without pause, slowly bend to your right side. Make sure your arms remain parallel. Hold for 5. Slowly straighten up.

Fig. 188 Now bend as far as possible to your left. Note that the arms remain parallel. This is a powerful stretch and must be accomplished gradually. Hold for 5. Slowly straighten up.

Fig. 189 Perform the extreme stretch on the right side. Hold for 5. Slowly straighten up.

Perform the entire routine of the Hip Bend twice. If you are attempting to reduce in the waist and hips, perform the entire routine up to five times.

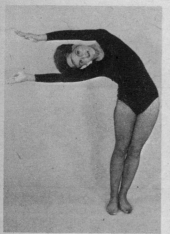
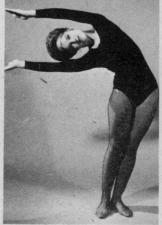

TRIANGLE POSTURE

Fig. 190 Assume the position illustrated. Note that the palms face downward and your legs are not too far apart.

Fig. 191 Slowly bend to the left side from your waist. Keep your knees straight. Rest your left hand on your knee and bring your right arm over as far as possible. Hold for 5.

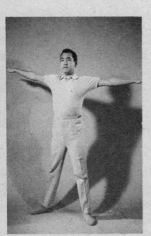
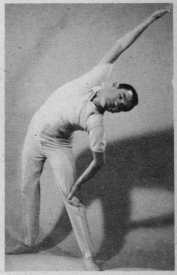

Fig. 192 Slowly straighten up and perform the identical movements to the right side. Remember to bring the arm over as far as possible. The elbow does not bend. Hold for 5.

Fig. 193 Slowly straighten up and assume a wider stance with the legs farther apart. Compare with *Fig. 190.*

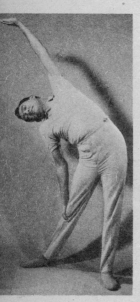

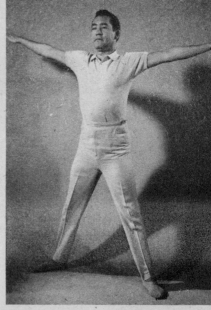

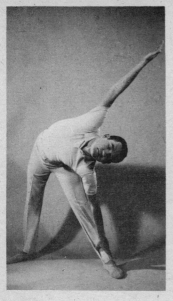
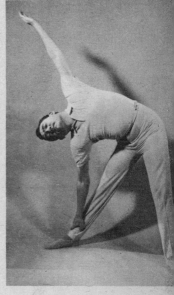

Fig. 194 Slowly bend to the left side and rest your hand as far down the leg as possible. The extreme position is to hold the ankle. The right arm comes far over. Hold for 5.

Fig. 195 Slowly straighten up and perform the identical movements to the right side. Note the various triangles that are formed with the limbs. Hold for 5. Slowly straighten up.

Perform the entire routine of the Triangle Posture twice. If you are attempting to reduce in the waist and hips, perform the entire routine up to five times.

LEG OVER

Fig. 196 In a lying position bend your right knee and raise the leg as illustrated.

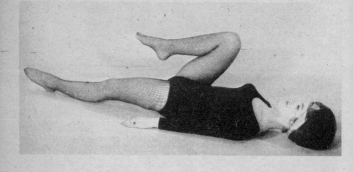

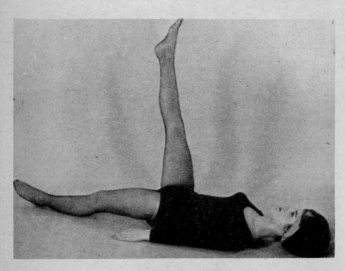

Fig. 197 Slowly straighten your right leg as illustrated.

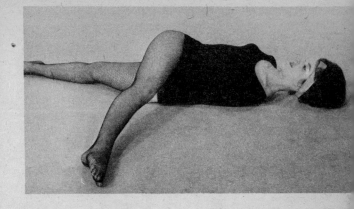

Fig. 198 Slowly bring the leg over and down to touch the floor if possible. You must keep both shoulders on the floor. Hold this position for a count of 10. Attempt to keep the right leg toward your head so that it makes a right angle with your body.

After the count of 10, slowly bring the right leg back, as in *Fig. 197*, and lower it to the floor. Perform the identical movements on the opposite side.

Fig. 199 The completed posture with the left leg. Note again that the leg is held high toward the head and that both shoulders remain on the floor. Hold for a count of 10. Bring the left leg back and slowly lower it to the floor. Repeat.

Perform the entire routine of the Leg Over exercise up to five times.

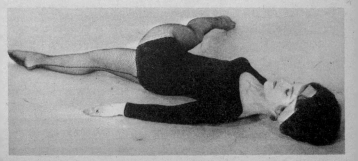

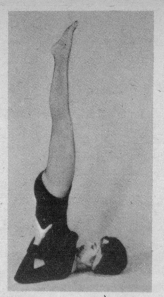

The Shoulder Stand is an important posture for Weight Control and the extreme position should be held for up to ten minutes whenever possible.

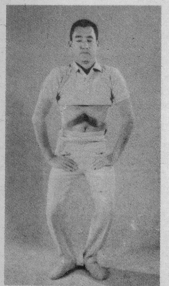

The excellent movements of the Abdominal Lift must certainly be included in the Weight Control routine; 100 to 200 movements and more are not excessive, when attempting to take off weight in the abdomen.

Posture

The sitting positions required of the sedentary worker will frequently result in habitually poor posture. Appearance and health are two aspects of the posture problem that should be considered by every worker who spends prolonged periods at a desk.

When we observe a person with poor posture, whose head is lowered, shoulders stooped and chest sunken, we associate this physical posture with age, fatigue and general oppression. Such a person seems to emit negative vibrations, and often just looking at him for a while can make us tired. Examine your own *natural* sitting and standing postures and determine if they need improvement. If so, it is well worth the effort to attempt improvement because a most pronounced change takes place when a person who has grown accustomed to stooped shoulders develops the ability to sit, stand and walk with an erect carriage. The entire body seems to awaken; the chest (which was forced to contract in the stooped posture) now expands naturally, appearance is greatly enhanced and a most important ability to breathe more fully develops. In a poor posture the abdomen will protrude; when the carriage is erect the abdominal area is naturally drawn in and organs that can be pushed out of position from a prolonged bad posture are relieved of this pressure. Also, many workers experience a continual vague discomfort in the shoulders, upper back and neck areas without realizing that this is the result of bad posture. An interesting psychological factor pertaining to this discussion is that a feeling of well-being and confidence seems to be related physically to a good carriage. You have possibly noticed that in moments of exceptional accomplishment or happiness there is an intensive physiological "lift" in the organism and a natural tendency to expand the chest and throw back the shoulders. It is not unreasonable to assume that we can reverse the process, that is, maintaining a good posture may be a type of *physical positive thinking*.

A good posture, however, cannot be forced or faked; it must be cultivated. If your posture is usually poor you may be able to stand erect for a few minutes when you want to make an impression or when you realize from time to time that your body is badly slumped. But you tire quickly in attempting to hold a good position for more than a short time, because the muscles involved are weak. In Yoga, we strengthen and rebuild the necessary muscles by working them in such a manner that the shoulders are systematically brought up and back through methodical movements. The two Yoga exercises that follow are recommended for the sedentary worker who wants to correct a posture problem. They not only require very little effort after the workday but actually provide a great relief from tension throughout the chest and shoulders.

In addition to these two fine, mild exercises, other important techniques to be practiced for a posture problem are: Bow, Backward Bend, Complete Breath, Arm and Leg Stretch, Locked Lotus.

POSTURE CLASP

Fig. 200   Sit in a cross-legged posture. Bring your left arm into the position illustrated. Note that the palm faces away from you.

Fig. 201   Bring your right hand over and lock the fingers.

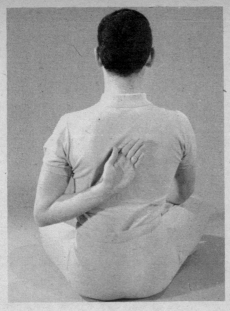

Fig. 200

Fig. 201

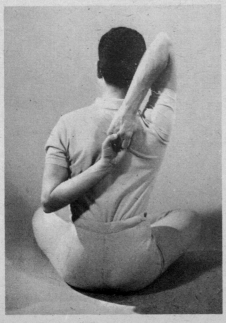

Fig. 202   Pull down with your left hand so that the right
arm is lowered several inches and a strong pull is felt
in your right shoulder. Hold for a count of 5.

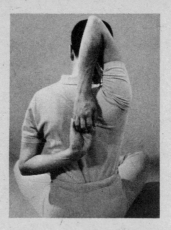

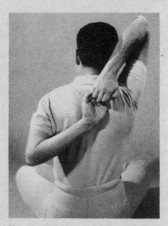

Fig. 203   Pull up with your right hand so that the left
arm is raised several inches and a strong pull is felt in
your left shoulder. Hold for 5. Repeat.

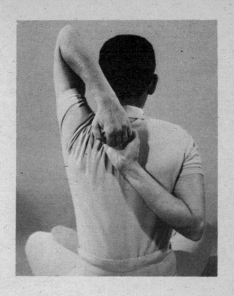

Fig. 204 Perform the identical movements on the opposite side.

Perform the up-and-down pulls twice on each side. Lock the fingers tightly. It is natural to feel tension in the arms.

ACTION AND BENEFITS OF THE POSTURE CLASP

The movements of this exercise are deceiving because they appear very simple but actually exert a great pull and loosening in vital areas of the upper arms and shoulders. You may have some difficulty in locking the fingers at first, but this will become possible after several attempts. The pulling up and down must be executed cautiously as you will realize that you are exercising the shoulder muscles in an unusual manner. Clasp the hands tightly together; this is good for firming and strengthening the arms.

MODIFIED CHEST EXPANSION

Fig. 205 Sit in a cross-legged posture and clasp your hands as illustrated.

Fig. 206 Raise your arms as high as possible without strain and slowly bend backward at the waist. The head drops backward also. Hold for a count of 5.

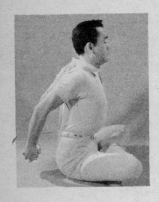

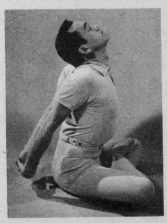

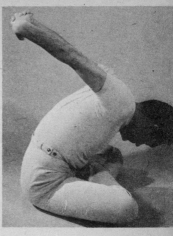

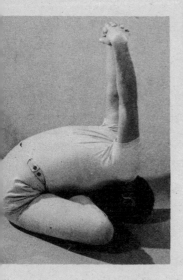

Fig. 207 Bend forward very slowly at the waist, keeping your arms high. Come forward as far as possible without strain. Hold for a count of 5. Slowly straighten up and repeat.

Fig. 208 The extreme position where the forehead rests on the floor. This position can be held for a count of 10 or longer, as it is extremely restful.

Perform the entire routine of the Modified Chest Expansion twice.

Headaches and Tension

In *Be Young with Yoga,* I described tension as the "Multi-Headed Dragon." I attempted to show the many forms tension may take and how it has become a fashionable scapegoat for our collective ills. It is a term used freely in all levels of our society to describe every imaginable affliction and is employed with exceptional skill by the advertising agencies. For purposes of our discussion, let us offer a generalized definition of tension (if the problem can be stated in simple terms we have a good chance to understand it and to cope with it). *Tension is a tightness or a squeezing which occurs in our organism mentally, emotionally and physically.* We "squeeze" ourselves at the point of tension. If you will observe yourself when you experience the feeling of tension (whether it be in your thoughts, emotions or body), you will become aware of this tightness or squeezing process. When you squeeze, you contract. The relief of this condition would obviously be to "de-contract," or, in other words, to *let go and relax.* There is no finer natural method than Yoga to effect this "de-contraction," to stop squeezing.

The sedentary worker is continually involved in many types of squeezing, of holding muscles tensed and contracted, of having to repress aggressive feelings, of forcing his mind to perform mechanical operations. Some of these situations cannot be avoided, but their negative impact can be greatly reduced. Many of these squeezings can be completely eliminated. One of the most prevalent symptoms of squeezing is the headache. A great deal of squeezing takes place in the head area, mentally and physically, but the headache is by no means caused only by tightness originating in the head. In the science of Yoga we know that the entire organism is so interrelated that an affliction in any area affects every other area in varying degrees. This is particularly true with the headache; it can be caused by such a multitude of things that we would be wise to learn and apply the "de-contraction" techniques rather than to seek the basic cause of the headache. We are emphasizing the headache because it is such a common problem among all sedentary workers, but remember that squeezing (almost all of which takes place unconsciously) results in tension that produces discomfort throughout the organism.

If you would like to become aware of just how much squeezing is actually transpiring unconsciously within you, try this experiment: Whenever you can remember to do so, observe yourself in action during the workday. "Freeze" in any of your working positions as you would stop a motion picture, then take stock of the way in which you are performing physically. Quickly run over your body with your mind, beginning with your toes and working rather rapidly upward. Note all of the muscles that are tensed needlessly, that is, muscles that are making no direct contribution to what you are doing at the moment. You will usually be astonished at the great amount of energy being wasted in this manner. As you observe the tensed muscles, it is necessary to issue a calm (not angry or stern) order to these muscles to relax. Often, simply observing that a muscle is contracted will automatically allow it to relax. By repeating this self-observation process often, you will find you habitually hold particular sets of muscles tensed. They may be in the legs, the stomach, the shoulders, the neck or other parts. With sufficient practice you will be able to change the pattern and habits of these muscles so that they "de-contract" when not in use. Physical "de-contraction" (which this book emphasizes) leads to emotional and mental relaxation. We hear a great deal these days about *psychosomatic* therapy in which the mind is used to influence the body. But the reverse is equally true and extremely important: The body influences the mind and the emotions in a most profound manner and is, in many ways, much easier to work with.

All of the Yoga techniques in this book will help you to stop squeezing. For the headache problem specifically, the inverted postures that bring the blood into the head, such as the Shoulder and Head Stands, seem to offer relief. Both techniques that follow have wonderful (and in many cases extraordinary) relaxation properties for the entire organism and offer immediate relief for a headache. (Recurring headaches should be dealt with by your physician.)

ALTERNATE NOSTRIL BREATHING

Fig. 209 Sit in a cross-legged posture. This breathing exercise is done in three parts: inhaling, retaining, exhaling. The flow of your breath is directed by stopping your nostrils alternately. Study the illustration for a moment and note carefully the position of the hand and fingers. Place the tip of your right thumb against your right nostril. Put your index and middle fingers together on your forehead. Place your ring and little fingers lightly against your left nostril. Keep your hand relaxed.

Fig. 210 Exhale completely through both nostrils. Close your *right* nostril by pressing your thumb against it, leaving your left nostril open. Inhale a slow, silent, complete breath through your *left* nostril in a rhythmic count of 8 beats.

Fig. 211 Keeping the right nostril pressed closed, now close the *left* nostril with the ring and little fingers as illustrated. Both nostrils are thus tightly closed and the breath is held for a rhythmic count of 4.

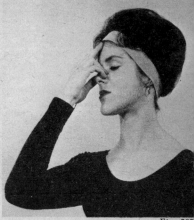

Fig. 209

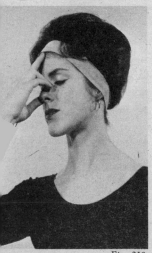

Fig. 210

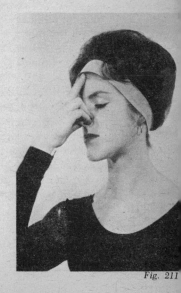

Fig. 211

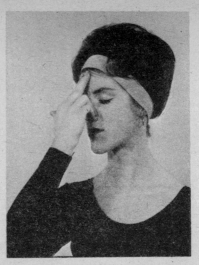

Fig. 212 Now remove the thumb from your *right* nostril (keeping the left pressed closed), and slowly and silently exhale fully through the *right* nostril in a rhythmic count of 8 beats.

When the air is completely exhaled from your lungs during the count of 8, without missing a beat in your rhythmic counting resume inhaling, this time through your *right* nostril (*the same nostril through which you just finished exhaling*). When the inhalation is completed during a rhythmic count of 8 beats, retain the air in your lungs by closing both nostrils as before during a rhythmic count of 4 beats. Then, without missing a beat, open your *left* nostril by removing the ring and little fingers and exhale completely through your left nostril during a rhythmic count of 8 beats (the *right* nostril remains closed). Without missing a beat in your counting begin the entire process again by inhaling through your *left* nostril, and so on.

Each time you return to the original point, that is, inhaling through the left nostril, you have completed *one round of* Alternate Nostril Breathing. You should perform five rounds of this exercise.

The following points should be carefully noted:

1 The counting for the breathing movements is rhythmic and continuous; 8-4-8; 8-4-8 and so on. Keep the beat going in your mind just like a metronome.
2 Attempt to inhale and exhale as quietly as possible. Try to avoid any hissing sound.
3 It will be somewhat difficult to perform the exhalation in the rhythmic count of 8; this will have to be pushed a little until you become accomplished.
4 Keep your eyes closed throughout the exercise.
5 Keep your hand relaxed, and try not to move your legs or body.

ACTION AND BENEFITS OF ALTERNATE NOSTRIL BREATHING

This is the third and final of our Yoga breathing techniques. It cannot be spoken of too highly. It will be appropriate at this point to delve a little more deeply into some of the underlying concepts of physical Yoga. *In the study of Yoga we can think of the functioning of the entire organism in all of its aspects (that is, physical, emotional and mental) as a continual interplay of positive and negative forces.* One of the universal principles upon which the study of all metaphysics has been based, and which may be observed throughout the entire history of the occult sciences, is this *positive-negative axiom.* The words *positive* and *negative* are used here in the way they are employed to explain many scientific phenomena.

Your body is always at work to keep a balance of the positive and negative forces in each of its functions. When either of these gets ahead of the other an abnormal physical, emotional or mental condition is produced. The Yogi will often diagnose an illness as an unbalancing of the positive-negative ratio. When this happens, the body draws upon all available sources of the life-force to restore the balance. A cure for an illness, or regaining a healthy, normal balance depends upon how serious the illness is and on how much life-force is available to combat it.

We have already called your attention to the fact that your breathing is directly connected with your thoughts and emotions. For example, if you are worried, fearful, anxious, depressed, excited, joyful, you will find that you tend to breathe rapidly and unevenly. On the other hand, when you are relaxed and calm, you will find that you tend to breathe more slowly and evenly. From this observation, the Yogis have established that reversing the process, that is, *controlling the breathing* in various ways, will calm the emotions and restore the positive-negative balance in the organism!

Another extremely interesting phenomenon that you can observe in your own breathing is that at any given time of the day or night the breath is flowing more strongly through one nostril than the other. This flow alternates between the nostrils, switching every few hours. This is one of nature's ways of regulating the balance of the positive and negative forces. See if you can observe the way this change occurs in your breathing during the period of one day. Because of this premise, the Yogi implies that the health of the organism can be affected if an individual has difficulty with one of his nostrils and continually breathes more fully through the other. The Alternate Nostril technique has helped many persons to correct this condition. It definitely seems to open the nostrils more fully.

As mentioned earlier, the physical aspect of Yoga (which is the primary concern of this book) is known in Sanskrit as "Hatha" Yoga. The word *Hatha* is derived from two Sanskrit roots: *Ha*, which means *sun* and *tha*, which means *moon*. These words have been symbolically applied by the Yogi to the nostrils, with the *right* nostril being named the *sun* channel or *positive* nostril and the *left* nostril the *moon* channel or *negative* nostril. Thus, the two nostrils are the main conductors of the positive and negative forces, dispersing these currents to every cell of the body. Similarly, physicists tell us that the brain generates an electrical current that is transmitted throughout the entire nervous system. Continuous production of this electricity seems to depend on a chemical process that takes place during the rhythmical action of breathing.

From Yoga we learn the relationship between the electrical current and the life-force; the positive charge comes from inhaling through the right nostril and the negative charge from the left. When this balance is upset, the body requires more of this electrical current and must take in more life-force from which to regulate the positive-negative ratio. This is why the breathing process accelerates under stress.

The word *Yoga* is derived from the Sanskrit root *yuj*, which means *join*. The words *Hatha Yoga* then, imply "the uniting or joining of the positive-negative currents." This joining enables one to experience an equilibrium, which in turn results in a state of unusual elevation of mind, body and spirit. One has only to perform the five rounds of this ancient technique exactly according to the given directions to experience the immediate results.

MODIFIED HEAD STAND

Fig. 213 Place your body in the position illustrated. Note the position of the toes. The top front of the head rests on the floor.

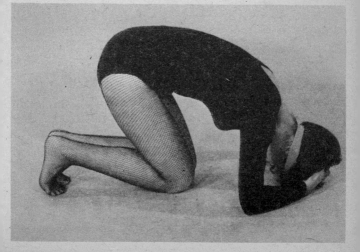

Fig. 214 Raise the body into the position illustrated. The idea is to get the blood into the head. If you are unable to execute the extreme arch as indicated, then any of the more modified positions will be adequate. Hold the position for one to three minutes, using a watch or clock for exact timing.

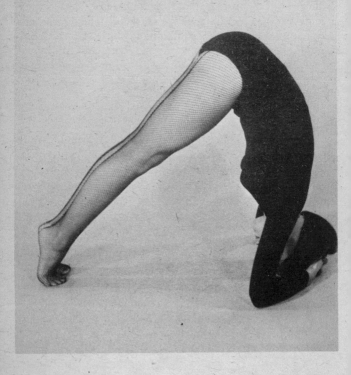

Constipation

Constipation is a serious and frequent problem of those who must spend a great deal of time in a sitting position. The peristaltic action of the intestines grows sluggish. The negative consequences reach into every aspect of the individual's life; it is unnecessary to elaborate on this fact. To cope with this problem it is obviously necessary to have a means of naturally stimulating the apparatus involved in the elimination process. Here again, we can appreciate the great ingenuity of the Yoga techniques because they provide us with the exercises needed for this natural stimulation. This has already been discussed in part under "Internal Exercising." Now we wish to concentrate on the intestines, colon, kidneys and the peristaltic action. We therefore employ not only the original Abdominal Lift, which we have already learned, but we add two additional positions, the Squatting and Sitting postures. We thus move the involved organs and glands into varying positions.

The number of lifts suggested in each of the three positions is for ordinary stimulation and to help prevent sluggishness. If there is a real problem, one must increase the number and perform several hundred, perhaps twice a day. These would be divided among the three positions. Several hundred or more lifts are not excessive nor do they require too much time to execute, once you become adept. With a few weeks' practice you will find you can execute up to twenty-five and more lifts with each exhalation, so that two or three hundreds lifts can be done within five to seven minutes. Naturally, in the case of a serious problem, one's physician should always be consulted before undertaking these suggestions.

The best time of the day to deal with sluggishness is upon arising. Drink four to six ounces of cool (not cold) water with a pinch of lemon. Allow a minute or two for the water to reach the stomach. Then begin the practice of the abdominal movements. Of course your diet plays an essential role in any constipation problem. If you are consuming more than the most moderate amounts of starches, sugars, refined, processed and fried foods (to name just a few of the offenders) you certainly increase the possibility of a constipation problem. A practical Yoga nutritional plan has been discussed in detail in my book *Be Young with Yoga*. I believe it is most important for the sedentary worker to realize that a laxative is an irritant and provides relief for a constipation problem because it causes a temporary abnormal condition with which the organism must cope. In coping with the irritation, temporary relief is afforded, but it must be obvious that relying on laxatives for regularity (and there are a great number of people who do) can only cause a constipation problem to become chronic eventually. The Yoga Abdominal Lifts provide the finest natural internal stimulation available.

SQUATTING ABDOMINAL LIFT

Fig. 215 Attempt to assume the squatting position illustrated. You will be sitting on your heels, your hands tightly gripping your knees. If you are unable to squat as indicated, rest your fingertips on the floor on either side. This helps to maintain your balance.

Now proceed to perform the movements exactly as described in the original Abdominal Lift. The lifts are intensified if you grip your knees very tightly. Attempt to perform three to five lifts with each exhalation. Repeat three to five times so that you execute twenty to twenty-five lifts in the squatting position.

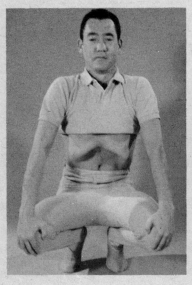
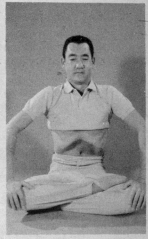

SITTING ABDOMINAL LIFT

Fig. 216 Sit in a cross-legged posture; rest your hands on your knees. Lean forward slightly and perform three to five lifts with each exhalation. Repeat three to five times so that you execute twenty to twenty-five lifts in the sitting position.

Exceptional Stiffness
and Arthritis

This is a vicious circle problem. Those whose spines, joints and limbs are unusually stiff are less inclined to exercise because of the acute discomfort involved—and the less inclined they are to exercise, the more inflexible they become. The seriousness of stiffness, as far as we are concerned in Yoga, cannot be overstated. It is the Yogic belief that the flow of life-force is greatly curtailed since "wherever you are stiff your energy is being sapped." Inhibiting the flow of life-force in the organism consequently results in many major and minor ills; therefore a stiff, tense body cannot possibly be a healthy one.

It is a tragic fact that at a relatively early age the sedentary worker who has a tendency toward stiffness resigns himself to it—and the thought of exercising to work out his spine, joints and limbs becomes more and more repugnant. This is completely understandable in light of the concept of calisthenic-type exercising, which so often leaves the body sore and aching. One who is exceptionally stiff will, naturally, have a great antipathy toward such movements. But we have an entirely different concept with Yoga because of the mild, methodical manipulation involved. There is no longer an excuse for any person to be unhealthily stiff, regardless of age or physical condition, once the Yoga techniques are undertaken seriously. This should encourage many sedentary workers who have for some time wanted to regain flexibility but have never been aware of how to proceed without experiencing the resulting discomfort of ordinary exercising.

The percentage of Yoga students who have reported to me that they have experienced a noticeable relief of their arthritic discomforts is extremely encouraging and cannot be ignored. As you probably know, arthritis victims seldom improve. They usually become worse. If they are fortunate, the pain may be kept to a minimum through medical treatment and the disease may be localized in one part of the organism. More often, however, arthritis *does* slowly spread, and the pain gradually becomes more intense. In other words, the chances for an arthritis cure by currently employed methods are extremely slim. It is our opinion (and this is based solely on extensive observation of students stricken with arthritis) that the one possibility which approaches a cure is the very patient and cautious self-manipulation of the body with emphasis on the joints. Notice that we stress *self*-manipulation, for while the various types of massage therapy and apparatus have proved helpful, they seem at best to offer only temporary relief. The term *self-manipulation* implies exercise and here again we encounter the dilemma of the vicious circle—the arthritis victim does not wish to exercise because his body hurts, but his body hurts more and more because he refuses to exercise. Again, this vicious circle can be broken with the Yogic movements, ideal for arthritis. I attribute the help the arthritis patient has received through Yoga to the *thoroughness* of the techniques. The slow-motion movements and the holds are able to reach deep into the joints. The methodical repetition of the movements, practiced very slowly and cautiously, seems within the course of time to produce wonderful results.

Whatever extreme position one is able to attain is held for increasing periods of time. If the student is able to move only one inch and hold a position for only five seconds, he is already beginning to exercise and manipulate. As a matter of fact, that is exactly how anyone with exceptional stiffness or arthritis should begin his manipulation of the afflicted areas. He should move only a few inches in any exercise until he begins to experience some discomfort. This extreme position should be held for a count of 5. He should attempt to repeat the movement two or three times. Each day he should attempt to move only an inch farther and hold one second longer, until he reaches a satisfactory distance and count. He should never strain, although there will probably be days in which he simply cannot practice at all. This is natural and to be expected. He must wait for a day or two until the intensely painful period has passed, then begin again. He can be encouraged by understanding that the bad spells are part of the system and that progress in cases of exceptional stiffness and arthritis is never in a straight line. One takes a few steps forward and one backward.

Another tragic aspect of arthritis is that this disease is by no means confined to the older individual. We find more and more younger people suffering from bone and joint pains. Scarcely a week passes that I do not receive letters complaining about arthritis from at least a half dozen sedentary workers who are not yet 35! My opinion is that this has been caused by insufficient exercising of the joints and improper diet. I believe that diet plays an extremely important role with regard to arthritis. Dairy foods seem to be among the chief offenders. I have observed that arthritic patients who have eliminated dairy foods from their diet (with the possible exception of moderate servings of nonfat milk and low-fat yogurt) have experienced noticeable relief from their symptoms. Many nutritionists are of the belief that dairy products are conducive to the formation of calcium deposits. Naturally, this differs with the individual, but it is certainly worthy of serious consideration by all who suffer from arthritis. A younger person who develops the first symptoms of arthritis (or any stiffness in the bones and joints) should be strongly encouraged to begin the Yoga exercises *immediately*. As always, all of the above statements are subject to the approval of one's physician.

We have already learned a number of important exercises for the joints. These include the Knee and Thigh Stretch for the knees, the Backward Bend for the toes and ankles, the Lotus Postures for the knees, ankles and feet, the Elbow Exercise for the elbow joints, the Shoulder Raise for the shoulder joints (bursitis), the Neck Twist and many exercises for the spine. The four techniques that follow are modified versions of exercises already learned. They illustrate how anyone can undertake the mild, nonstrenuous and progressive practice of not only these, but all of the Yoga postures.

MODIFIED LEG PULL

Fig. 217 A very mild pull for the legs and back. One attempts to hold only the knees (or thighs if necessary) and to perform a moderate pull forward. A count of 5 to 10 is sufficient.

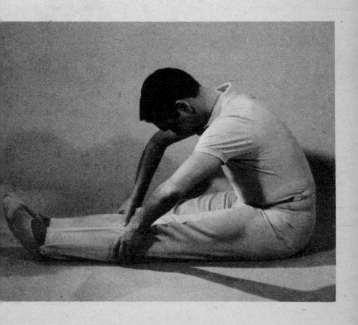

MODIFIED COBRA

Fig. 218 The hands are placed beneath the shoulders at the very beginning of the exercise and are used continually for the cautious pushing up of the trunk. The trunk is raised very carefully only a moderate distance. Hold for five to ten seconds.

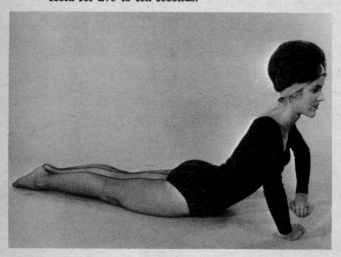

MODIFIED TOE AND FOOT EXERCISE

Fig. 219 The buttocks are lowered very slowly onto the heels while the toes rest on the floor as depicted. The fingers provide support so that the amount of weight placed on the heels can be completely controlled. Each day a little more weight can be supported. The hold can be from one to twenty seconds. This movement is preparatory for the Backward Bend and can also be practiced with the feet on the floor, rather than the toes.

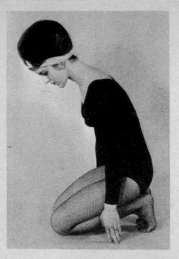

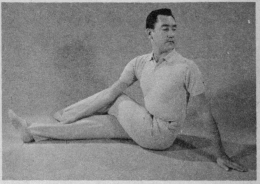

MODIFIED TWIST

Fig. 220 An easy form for the twisting movements of the Full Twist and the Simple Twist. Here the leg that is crossed over is stretched far out so that the arm can easily take hold of the calf. The opposite hand remains resting flat on the floor and the trunk may be twisted with any degree of intensity desired. Compare this modified exercise with the Full Twist. The position may be held for five to ten seconds and repeated three times. It is then performed on the opposite side.

Insomnia

The sedentary worker is much more likely to be plagued with insomnia than the manual, active worker. This is particularly true of those in various executive capacities and the worker who has added responsibilities, such as the supervision of others. It is also a problem that besets creative people who work primarily with ideas. The worries and concerns of the workday refuse to vanish as one departs from the office or studio and are often taken home and to bed. Of course the insomnia problem is certainly not confined to those described. Anyone can have insomnia for any reason and suffer from one night to twenty years! Generally speaking, however, we have found that among the students in our classes, those whose work is of a physically active nature are less likely to have insomnia than those whose professions are predominantly in the realm of thoughts, ideas and calculations. The reason for this is obvious: If the body is truly tired, the organism will be forced into sleep. The inactive, sedentary worker is not genuinely tired but *depleted* in a peculiar manner: Tension has built up throughout his body and the phonograph record that has been set going in his mind during the day, and that has exhausted the brain, continues to play over and over far into the night.

There is a difference between a serious problem that has a great impact upon the organism because of a genuine threat (and hence demands continual attention making sleep difficult) and a vague physical and mental "gnawing" which, almost mechanical in nature, keeps the victim awake perhaps one or two nights a week, or possibly more. The former can be *dealt with directly because it is real.* In the spiritual aspect of Yoga such problems are understood in a certain philosophical context. (This is an additional study and cannot be presented in the necessary detail in this discussion.) Nonetheless, the serious, real problem is sooner or later dealt with in one form or another and thus poses much less of a dilemma than the vague anxiety which continues to gnaw night after night, week after week and, often, year after year. For the latter type of problem, great relief is offered through the Yoga techniques. The problem, as many of those we have already discussed, appears to be twofold, that is, mental (in this case a repetition of meaningless thought forms) and physical (tension and restlessness). We use the word *appears* above because we have learned that in Yoga the physical and mental are not separate but completely interdependent. But one must be continually reminded of this vital physical-mental relationship, because most of the time we seem to live (exist and function) in the brain *or* in the body. We are seldom fully aware of ourselves as an *integrated psychosomatic entity.* It is a major objective of Yoga to bring about this realization.

We have found that a particular routine of the physical techniques, performed just before retiring, not only helps eliminate the tension in key muscles and joints but reduces the mental "squeezing" that perpetuates the restlessness of the mind. This routine is presented below.

In answer to the frequent question, "How much sleep is sufficient?" we can only say, "Only *you* know, because each of us is different in his requirements." Some can live their entire lives with six hours or less of sleep nightly. Most require eight, nine or even ten hours. If you sleep eight hours and are tired when you awaken, you either have not had enough sleep or have slept poorly. The more toxic the body, the more sleep required, because nature attempts to eliminate toxins as well as to rebuild during sleep. You will find that if you are eating sensibly and practicing your Yoga exercises, your body generally requires less sleep. The earlier you retire, the more value your sleep will have. Retiring *after* midnight, if you must arise early for work, is a most injurious habit and can shorten your life. Insufficient sleep will certainly make you irritable and jumpy; it is a recognized fact that lack of sleep is one of the surest ways to break down the nervous system.

The yawn is nature's indication that you need to rest or sleep. When you begin to yawn in the evening hours, no matter what the hour, your body and brain will no longer be able to function at their best, and it is time for sleep. Work done while yawning is subject to numerous errors. If you want to reduce the possibility of insomnia to a minimum, make certain that *you do not eat for at least ninety minutes before going to bed*. This includes hot milk, tea and other concoctions believed to induce sleep. Your body does not want to have to go through the digestive process when it should be preparing for a sound sleep. The sleeping surface should offer some resistance; you should not sink into your mattress. Some students have found that dispensing with a pillow and sleeping without the head raised helped them to feel more alive and rested in the morning. You might like to experiment with this idea.

There are only four techniques in the Insomnia Routine. These are to be practiced as follows: Cobra, perform twice as instructed; Neck Twist, perform once in each of the three positions; Alternate Leg Pull, perform twice with each leg; Alternate Nostril Breathing, perform five rounds as instructed.

Some students find it expedient to do most of their Yoga practicing before retiring. Others find that this is overly stimulating and releases a great deal of energy, making sleep difficult. Again, this is a highly individual matter, and you must experiment to determine your own reaction to the various possibilities of practice.

Poor Breathing;
Exercises with Breathing

Three essential aspects of Yogic breathing have been discussed in the three breathing techniques already learned. These were: Complete Breath, Charging Breath and Alternate Nostril Breathing. Because of the importance and profundity of the Yogic breathing concept we suggest that you reread the text of these three exercises often. It is hoped that you will be sufficiently impressed to pay increasing attention to the breathing process and the incredible manner in which it sustains and controls life. We know that with the Complete Breath we can improve the quality of the blood; we know that we can revitalize and cleanse with the Charging Breath; the Alternate Nostril Breathing is unsurpassed for a natural tranquilizer.

In more advanced Yoga, breathing plays an increasingly important role. Specifically, the breath is taken at the start of almost all exercises and the *retention* is gradually increased. The objective is to stimulate and awaken more and more of the potential vital force that lies asleep within the organism. Toward this end the breath (which is the awakening power) is retained longer and longer until a minute or more is spent in each position. In the ultimate stages of advanced Hatha Yoga the student, under prolonged and careful guidance of the master (*guru*), is taught how breath may actually be suspended. For our purposes we can make use of the breath retention practice in a very mild manner and derive excellent results.

We have already practiced some breath retention in the Chest Expansion and Alternate Nostril Breathing. When you feel that you have become proficient in most of the exercises (this should require quite some weeks or even months, depending on your physical condition when you begin) and that the more extreme positions are accomplished with relative ease, you can begin the breath retention in conjunction with each of the exercises. The procedure is as follows: You begin the inhalation as you begin the physical movements of the exercise. The inhalation is completed by the time you are ready for the stretch. The breath is at first retained for five seconds, then gradually worked up to ten seconds. In certain exercises, a retention of five to ten seconds is sufficient to complete the stretching portion; in other exercises a retention of five to ten seconds will take you only partially through the holding position. Therefore, either you will be exhaling as you come out of the stretch or you will exhale and maintain the holding position until the necessary count is completed. For example, in the Preliminary Leg Pull, you perform a slow inhalation as you raise your arms and lean backward (depicted in *Figs.* 2 and 3). In practicing breath retention you would then retain the breath as you come forward, grasp your legs and pull your trunk downward. You could probably retain your breath through the movements of *Figs.* 4-8. If so, you would gently and quietly exhale as you slowly straighten up, pause and rest a few moments, then start another inhalation as you bring up your arms to repeat the movements. If you were unable to comfortably retain your breath throughout the movements of *Figs.* 4-8, you would simply exhale slowly and quietly whenever necessary, but you would continue the physical movements breathing normally. *You must never, under any circumstances, hold your breath one moment longer than you feel completely comfortable doing so.* If any discomfort or dizziness is experienced, discontinue the breath retention for several days, then try again cautiously. The inhalation is a form of the Complete Breath; that is, it is a very deep type of breathing with the abdomen distended and the chest expanded whenever possible.

In an exercise such as the Cobra, you would perform the inhalation while in the position of *Fig. 9,* then retain the breath for approximately ten seconds. This would take you partially through the raising movements of *Figs. 10* and *11,* and possibly *12.* You would then exhale but continue with the exercise, breathing normally.

In the Bow, you would first perform all of the physical movements necessary to prepare for the extreme position. These would be the movements of *Figs. 17* and *18.* While in the position of *Fig. 18* you would execute the inhalation and retain during the extreme positions of *Figs. 19* and *20,* then exhale during the movements of *Figs. 21-23.* With a little practice you will quickly determine where the inhalation, retention and exhalation should occur in each exercise.

It is not necessary to retain the breath with each exercise. This sometimes proves tiring. You can choose several of the postures for breath retention during each practice period. For the sedentary worker and for anyone whose breathing habits are poor (shallow, erratic) from congestion, smog, smoking, air-conditioning, respiratory trouble and so forth, this type of mild Yogic breath retention should prove most beneficial.

Part Four

Yoga for the Housewife

The sedentary worker knows that he is deficient in the exercise department because he is able to feel the results of his inactivity. The housewife is the supreme example of the person who believes she is getting all the exercise she needs—indeed, her complaint is that she usually gets a lot more than she needs. But the fact is that as a group, housewives are seriously deficient in true exercising (often more so than the sedentary workers because of the nature of housework). The housewife confuses the *amount* of activity with the *type* of activity. She fails to distinguish between just plain activity (housework) and the systematic manipulation of the body that is true exercise. The duties of the housewife *promote* conditions of physical and emotional stress, and it is therefore essential that she take the time to relieve this stress through proper exercising. If the activities of housework (cleaning, shopping, child care and so forth) constituted true exercise, then we would not see the housewife tense, irritable, overweight, flabby, depressed and complaining of every type of soreness and pain.

Housework, and all that it entails, is not fun, but it *is* the work of the housewife. As such, it is important and must be done with a sense of fulfillment and satisfaction. To work is a privilege, and through it inner growth and self-development take place. If the housewife does not experience such satisfaction from her work, if housework is continual drudgery and not meaningful, then she eventually becomes irritable (frustrated), morbid and otherwise depressed. This is passed on to other members of the household and can make for very unhappy living. We all know how prevalent such a condition is in many homes. No one can deny or lessen the responsibilities and pressures under which the housewife works. The point is, she must be up to these pressures day after day, and she often needs more continuous, sustaining energy than her husband at the office. To do her work well she must *feel* well and *look* well. When her physical and psychological conditions are healthy, the housewife takes pleasure and finds meaning in her work.

A series of Yoga exercises specifically for the housewife will impart energy, offer relaxation when needed and provide a firm, streamlined body. This series is presented in the following pages. Some of the techniques are additions to and variations of exercises offered earlier for the sedentary worker. The housewife may perform some or all of these previous exercises, but if this is impractical, she should definitely practice the routine which follows. This routine has been devised with many of the specific problems of the housewife considered, such as the strain which results from her various bending and stooping positions and the need for firming, streamlining and relatively quick relief from emotional strain.

The exercises may be practiced at any convenient time of the day. Many housewives found that practicing the exercises with my morning television program (after the children and husband had left the house) gave them energy and an elevated feeling that was sustained for many hours. But choose the time of the day most convenient for you. It is a good practice to choose the same time each day if possible, because then the idea becomes a habit. Of course the following exercises are not limited solely to the housewife; the techniques and variations can be incorporated into the practice of the sedentary worker.

Two additional important tips for the housewife: (1) Stretch often during your housework; (2) Make it a rule always to move with grace, regardless of how mundane you may think your activities are. If you begin to create a ballet (longer, smoother arm, leg and trunk movements) out of sweeping, cleaning and the like, you may laugh at first but you will be surprised at how quickly your body assumes added poise and grace and at how good this makes you feel. Don't be afraid to exaggerate these movements; you will see how quickly your increased poise will lend added beauty to your body and how this is noticed by everyone who knows you. Also, several times a day, "freeze" your body when you find yourself in a bending, stooping or reaching position, then proceed to stretch your body to and fro from whatever position you are in. Stretching removes tension and releases energy—and this is what the housewife needs desperately!

OVERHEAD SQUAT

Fig. 221 In a standing position place your palms together and rest the hands on your head as illustrated. Note the symmetry of the arms.

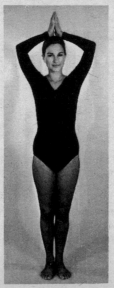

Fig. 222 In very slow motion bend your knees and lower your body.

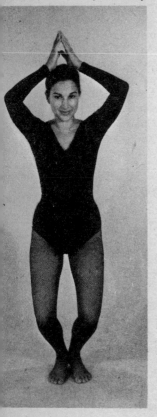
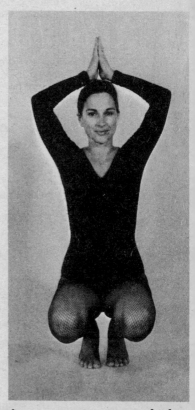

Fig. 223 Continue until you are resting on your heels. There is no hold in this exercise. Begin immediately to push up *very slowly*, staying on your toes all the way.

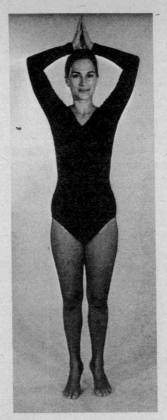

Fig. 224 Raise the body until you are on the tips of the toes as illustrated. Then rest the entire foot on the floor, as in *Fig. 221*. Without pause, repeat.

Perform the Overhead Squat five times. This exercise for firming and strengthening the legs is designed to impart balance, grace and poise in ballet-type movements. Attempt to feel the beauty and symmetry of your body as it executes these movements. Also note the repetition in the directions of the word *slowly*. This is not a quick, calisthenic-type "deep knee bend."

SEATED SIDE BEND

Fig. 225 Sit as illustrated. The fingers are interlaced behind the head.

Fig. 226 Very slowly bend as far as possible to your left, pointing the left elbow toward the floor. The illustration depicts a beginning position; gradually the elbow should touch the floor (see *Fig. 230*). Hold your extreme position for a count of 5. Keep both knees close to the floor.

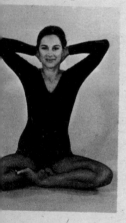

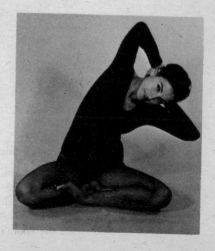

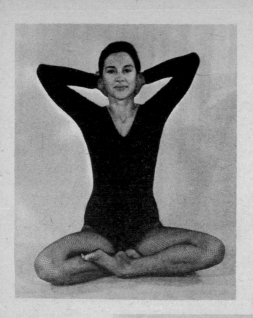

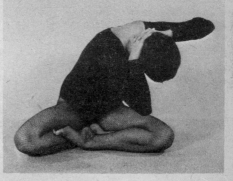

Fig. 227 Very slowly and gracefully straighten up.

Fig. 228 Now twist your trunk to the left and slowly bring your right elbow down toward your left knee. The illustration depicts a moderate position; gradually the elbow should touch the knee (see *Fig. 232*). Keep your knees close to the floor. Hold for a count of 5.

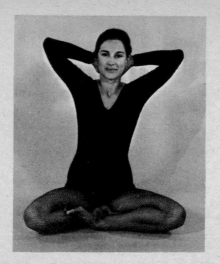

Fig. 229 Very slowly straighten up.

Fig. 230 Now perform the same movements to the right side. Very slowly bend at the waist and lower the right elbow as far as possible. Hold for 5.

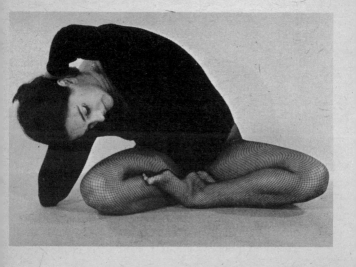

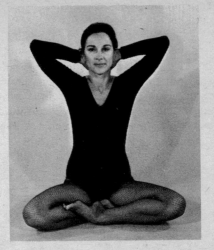

Fig. 231 Very slowly straighten up.

Fig. 232 Twist your trunk to the right, and slowly bring your left elbow down to the right knee. Hold for 5. Slowly straighten up and repeat the entire routine.

Perform the entire routine of the Seated Side Bend three times. This is an excellent exercise for flexibility, firming and reducing inches throughout the waist and hips. The movements must be performed with grace and poise so that the exercise takes on the appearance of a seated ballet.

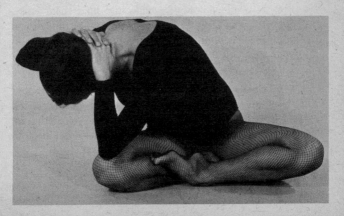

LION

Fig. 233 Sit with your legs folded beneath you so that
your heels are against the buttocks and your knees are
together on the floor. Your weight is on your heels exactly as in the first part of the Backward Bend. Rest
your hands on your knees, palms downward.

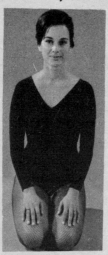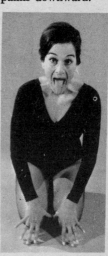

Fig. 234 Move your trunk forward, open your eyes as
wide as possible, tense your muscles throughout the
body, spread your fingers wide and hold them tense,
stick out your tongue as far as it can go—as though you
would touch your chin with it. Feel every muscle in
your face and neck become tense. Hold for a count of
15.

Very slowly bring the tongue back into the mouth and
simultaneously allow all muscles to relax. Settle back
on your heels as in *Fig.* 233. Make sure you withdraw
very slowly, like a cat slowly settles back after stretching. Relax for a few moments and repeat.

Perform the Lion three times and count 15 in the extreme position. People with special problems pertaining to the face, chin, neck or throat may perform the Lion five times and hold the extreme position up to one full minute.

ACTION AND BENEFITS OF THE LION

The Lion has the ability to relieve tension and acts as an excellent toning and refresher technique. Every housewife has need of such an exercise several times each day. With the Lion we are able to exercise and stimulate areas of the face, throat and neck that we are unable to reach in our ordinary activities or exercises.

Most people, as they grow older, seem to believe that it is perfectly natural to have wrinkles, double chins, sagging skin in the throat area and voices which grow increasingly harsh and pinched. They attribute these symptoms, with many other troubles, to the convenient scapegoat of "growing older." But as already pointed out, the Yogi refutes this idea because he does not believe in the common concept of old age. He maintains that areas of the body that are suffering from premature aging are generally not receiving proper nourishment from the blood (poor circulation) and are lacking the necessary stimulation and muscular toning.

If you did not use your arm for a prolonged period of time, the muscles would lose their tone and the flesh on your arm would begin to wither and sag. If the skin around your neck and face is sagging, your neck and face muscles have lost their resilience due to lack of exercise and are too weak to support this skin. No cream, powder, lotion, oil, machine or massage is going to restore the tone of face or neck muscles, *but you can begin to do so yourself from within.* Specifically, we make the following claims for the Lion exercise: It helps to prevent sagging face and neck muscles, improves the appearance of the skin by aiding circulation in the face area, will often reduce wrinkles and crow's feet in the eye area, massages the larynx, improves the quality of the voice, will help to relieve a sore throat. You may be surprised that such claims can be made for the apparently simple movement of sticking out your tongue. But it is very easy to test these claims; just give the technique a fair trial as directed. You have only to try the movements of the Lion a few times to realize that in no way can you feel the muscles of your eyes, face, chin and neck being stretched and exercised so strongly. You will feel how the blood is brought into these areas and how the relief of tension leaves the face feeling toned and refreshed.

Do not be afraid to stick your tongue out as far as you can and to make a ferocious face, because the greater the stretch the more benefit usually derived. Remember to assume all of the ferocity of a lion about to pounce. Feel every muscle in your neck and face grow tense during the posture; hold the eyes wide (to exercise the surrounding area) and spread the fingers as far apart as possible (to strengthen them). Relax all of your muscles very slowly upon completion of each extreme position, and you will feel the warmth in the facial area as the blood flows into it.

The housewife can perform the Lion several times a day— seated or standing at anytime she wishes to exercise the facial muscles. The sedentary worker needs privacy for the Lion and usually must wait for her (or his) regular Yoga practice period at home. One's fellow workers are inclined to take a dim view of the Lion practiced at the office.

COBRA TWIST

These additional movements are added to the Cobra, which has already been learned. They are excellent for the housewife whose work requires a great deal of bending and stooping.

Fig. 235 Here is the completed posture of *Fig. 13*. We continue from this position, after the count of 10 is concluded.

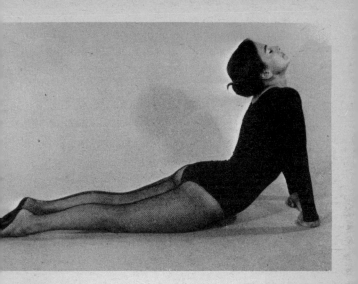

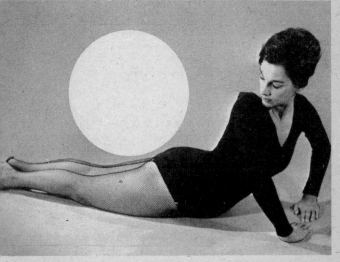

Fig. 236 Very slowly bend your elbows slightly so that you can twist your trunk, and turn your head until you can see your right heel. Hold for a count of 5.

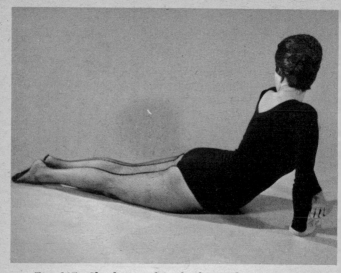

Fig. 237 Slowly straighten back into the position of *Fig. 235* and perform the identical twist to the left. Hold for 5. Straighten up and continue with the exercise by lowering the trunk as directed in *Figs. 14, 15* and *16*.

ROCKING BOW

These additional movements are added to the Bow, which has already been learned. They are designed to place emphasis on the lumbar area, where many housewives experience great discomfort from bending.

Fig. 238 This is the completed Bow posture of *Fig. 20*. We continue from this position after the count of 10 is concluded.

Fig. 239 In the next two movements we attempt a hobbyhorse-type rocking on the abdomen. This continuous rocking movement is performed very slowly, without pause. *Fig. 239* depicts the forward movement of the rocking.

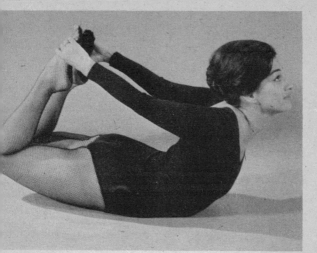

Fig. 238

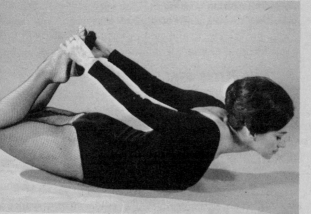

Fig. 239

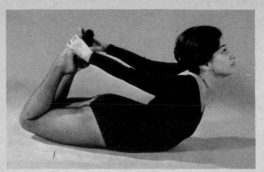

Fig. 240   Here is the backward movement, in which the trunk is brought up and back as far as possible without strain. Notice the head is held high. You will feel an intensive strengthening in the lower back. Try to keep your knees together.

Perform the rocking movements five times. Even if you are able to move only several inches you will benefit greatly. The movements must be performed with slowness and caution because they are very powerful. When the five rocking movements are completed, continue with the exercise as directed in *Figs. 21, 22* and *23*.

SHOULDER STAND VARIATIONS

These additional movements are added to the Shoulder Stand, which has already been learned. They are designed to relieve pressure and tension that builds in the legs from prolonged periods of standing while cooking, ironing, cleaning and so forth.

Fig. 241   This is the completed Shoulder Stand posture of *Fig. 117*. We continue the movements from this position after you have concluded your count of one to three minutes.

Fig. 242   Perform a slow split with your legs and move them apart as far as possible. Hold for a count of 10.

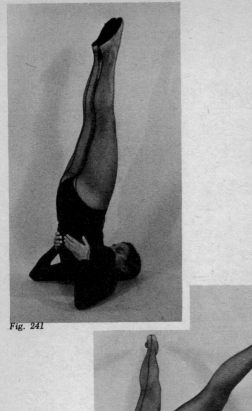

Fig. 241

Fig. 242

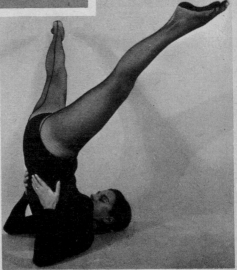

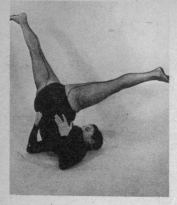

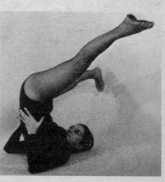

Fig. 243 Now keeping the legs apart, perform a slow twisting movement with your trunk to the left. The trunk twists, not the legs. Hold for 10.

Fig. 244 Keeping the legs apart, perform a slow twist to the right. Remember that it is the trunk that twists, not the legs. Hold for 10.

Return to the position of *Fig. 242* and slowly straighten once again into the position of *Fig. 241*. Then continue with the exercise by coming out of the extreme position as described in *Figs. 118, 119* and *120*.

ALL FOURS ABDOMINAL LIFT

This position is added by the housewife to the Abdominal Lifts already learned. This exercise is exceptionally valuable for new mothers to help restore organs to their proper positions.

> *Fig. 245* Place your body in the all-fours position as illustrated. The knees are close together and the arms parallel.

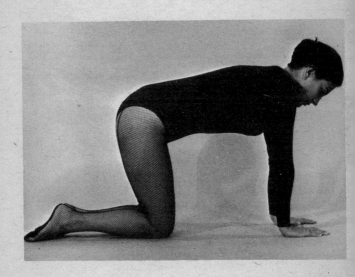

Fig. 246 The movements of the Abdominal Lifts already learned are now performed. It is difficult to depict in this illustration, but the lift is being performed, and the cavity which is formed is just as great as that of *Figs. 154, 215* and *216*. Perform as many lifts as possible with the exhalation. Sit back on your heels and relax a moment. Resume the all-fours position and repeat.

Perform three to five times, attempting to execute approximately ten lifts with each exhalation.

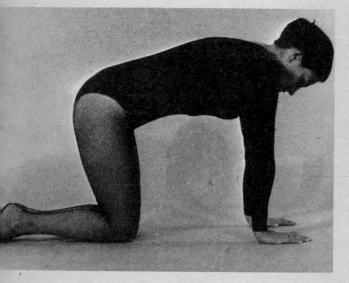

CORPSE POSTURE

This is a technique designed to refresh and revitalize. One of the most ancient of all relaxation exercises, it is a must for every housewife who would retreat for a few minutes from the activities of the household.

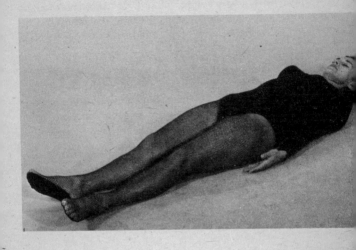

Fig. 247 Lie as illustrated. Actually, the illustration depicts the final objective of the technique, which is *complete and deep relaxation*. This is achieved as follows: Close your eyes and place your consciousness on the tips of the toes. Gradually draw your consciousness through the foot, ankle, calf, knee, thigh, and so on. As you intently feel each of these areas, issue a firm but calm order that all of the muscles in these areas must relax completely. Continue to draw your consciousness through the torso and the neck. *Remember, this is performed very slowly.* When you reach the neck area, place the consciousness through the arms. When you reach the neck, your body will be completely relaxed. Concentrate next on the face and have these muscles

relax. Then spend approximately one minute attempting to see (with your mind's eye) your entire organism filled with a very bright, white light. Allow no thought to occupy your mind; visualize only the bright, white light. No matter how often it fades, or disappears altogether, continue to bring it back.

This technique should require approximately three minutes to be performed slowly and correctly. Along with Alternate Nostril Breathing, the Corpse Posture is wonderful for calming the organism after emotional and mental disturbances.

Part Five

Advanced Positions

A satisfactory position of almost all Yoga exercises can be achieved within a few weeks of practice. At the end of several months you will feel as though you have been practicing Yoga all of your life. The exercises will be second nature and most of the movements will seem as natural as walking. Students usually find themselves so limber and accomplished that they seek more of a challenge from the postures—and Yoga is happy to oblige.

There are hundreds of different Yoga postures. Many of them represent astonishing dexterity of the spine and limbs that has been accomplished after long years of practice. Such advanced postures are sometimes depicted in Hatha Yoga books and demonstrated by visiting Yogis from India. This is often unfortunate, since such postures not only are impractical and unnecessary for the average person of the western world, but they have a most discouraging effect on many people and prevent them from ever getting started. For example, a 70-year-old grandmother who leafs through a book on Yoga and sees a supple, young Hindu executing a Full-Lotus in the Head Stand, cannot readily imagine her stiff, tense body in this posture. Assuming that such a posture must be part of the necessary achievement to gain benefit from the Yoga study, she will naturally pursue the idea no further. Actually, as I trust I have shown in this book, such a woman could derive great benefits from the Yoga exercises, following the outline and instructions as presented in the section dealing with "Excessive Stiffness."

The advanced Yoga postures (which should always be identified as "advanced" in all treatises and demonstrations) are extremely meaningful and have great value when a certain stage of study is reached. If and when you reach such a stage and are determined to continue, you cannot help but find the path. This is a law of Yoga. You will then, under the close supervision of a master, engage in many practices for purposes of cleansing and stimulating that, in former years, you would have found "weird" and seemingly without meaning. It is this type of advanced practice which has, through various means, filtered into sensational newspaper and magazine articles, radio and television programs and given rise to the tragically distorted concept of Yoga held by so many people in the western world.

It is important also, for purposes of clarification, to understand that those groups of peoples of the Far and Near East who do strange things such as walking on hot coals, sticking needles into their bodies, allowing themselves to be "buried alive" and so forth are known as "Fakirs" and are never to be confused with the Yogi. Fakirs are not fakers. They are actually able, through self-hypnosis, to perform extraordinary feats such as those mentioned. They do so for alms, food and favors. But the Fakir is not a Yogi. Comic strips, radio, movies, television and other media have contributed to the confusion by often referring to Fakirs as "Yogis." One who practices Yoga will never permit anything unnatural or harmful to be done to his body or mind. Every movement and aspect of the science of Yoga is completely natural and *for purposes of development of human potential.* Psychic or occult phenomena, so-called extrasensory perception (ESP), levitation and so forth are considered *obstructions to the objectives of Yoga and are never tolerated by the guru.* Although Yogis do gain extraordinary power and control, they are not interested in their powers as an end in themselves and will employ such powers only under most unusual circumstances.

All of the exercises presented in this book must, of necessity, be completely practical. The very difficult postures—those that I know require long periods of time to perfect—will not be included here. The advanced exercises that *are* offered in the following pages are the very extreme positions of techniques already learned. Your body will tell you when you are ready to attempt these extreme positions (of course there is increased value to be derived from them). Always proceed very cautiously, since the extreme positions make intense demands on the organism. You will feel a wonderful sense of accomplishment as you gradually succeed.

EXTREME CHEST EXPANSION

Fig. 248 This is a continuation of the backward bend movement in *Fig. 159* of the Chest Expansion. Sufficient flexibility has now been gained so that the thumbs of the clasped hands are braced against the backs of the thighs and a more intensive backward stretch is performed. The eyes should be kept open; the breath should *not* be held in the extreme position. You should not attempt this movement until your spine feels extremely flexible. Hold for a count of 5.

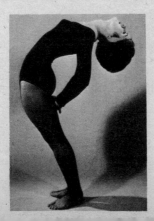

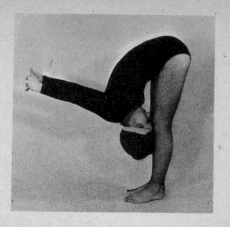

Fig. 249 The extreme forward bend (compare with *Fig. 161* of the Chest Expansion). The spine is now flexible enough so that the forehead can rest on the knees. Note how far down the arms have come and the over-all beauty of the figure. Hold for a count of 10.

Continue with the exercise as described in *Figs. 162* and *163*.

EXTREME ALTERNATE LEG PULL

Fig. 250 This is the same position as depicted in *Fig. 55* of the Alternate Leg Pull. The extreme position is attempted after a count of 30 in this position.

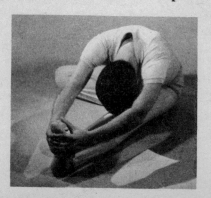

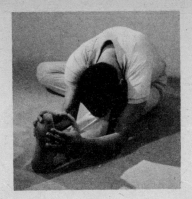

Fig. 251 The fingers now hold the toes, and the elbows are lowered to touch the floor on either side of the leg. This represents the ultimate stretching and firming for the calf. Hold this extreme position for a count of 10. Perform the identical movements with the right leg.

The extreme position of *Fig. 251* is added to the advanced position of *Fig. 250*. Note that the advanced position is held for thirty seconds but the extreme position for only ten. The movements are performed twice with each leg.

EXTREME COMPLETE LEG PULL

Fig. 252 This is the same position as depicted in *Fig. 60* of the Complete Leg Pull. The extreme position is attempted after a count of 30 in this position.

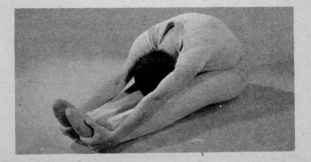

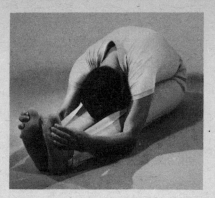

Fig. 253 The fingers now hold the toes of both feet, and the elbows are lowered to touch the floor at the sides. This position represents an extreme stretching and firming for both legs and the entire back. Hold this extreme position for a count of 10.

The extreme position of *Fig. 253* (held ten seconds) is added to the position of *Fig. 252* (held for thirty seconds).

Once you have accomplished the first position of the Plough you are ready to practice the two positions which follow. You must be able to rest your feet on the floor, as seen in *Fig. 39*, or you will be unable to proceed with these advanced postures.

2nd PLOUGH POSITION

Fig. 254 Proceed from *Fig. 39* after a count of 10 as instructed. Bring your hands up and clasp them on the top of your head. Your arms bend at the elbows and rest on the floor. This change of the arm position will allow you to push your toes several inches farther back, so that you will feel the pressure working up through the *middle* area of your back. (Compare *Figs. 39* and *254* to note the extra distance.) Keep your eyes closed; do not bend your knees; attempt to breathe as slowly as possible. Hold for a count of 10.

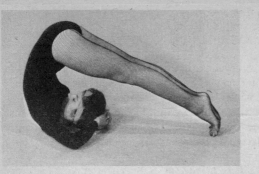

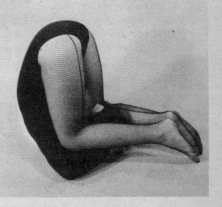

3rd PLOUGH POSITION

Fig. 255 Proceed from *Fig. 254* after the count of 10 is completed. Bend your knees and try to lower them to rest on either side of your head. The knees can fit inside the bent arms. The pressure is now on the extreme upper back and the cervical vertebrae. Attempt to breathe as slowly as possible. Hold for a count of 10.

The entire Plough routine is performed twice and each of the three positions held for a count of 10. To come out of the third Plough Position, place your arms back down on the floor and proceed to roll forward as instructed in *Figs. 40-43.*

EXTREME BACKWARD BEND

Once you have accomplished the completed Backward Bend posture on your toes (*Fig. 78*) you should slowly and cautiously attempt the very advanced position which follows. There is a great sense of accomplishment and satisfaction that comes from achieving this posture and if one works patiently and progressively, he can usually succeed.

Fig. 256   This movement is begun after you feel very secure in the position of *Fig. 78*. Very slowly and cautiously, bend your right elbow and attempt to gradually lower it to the floor. You must feel no strain, and you may only be able to lower the elbow a few inches for many weeks. The moment you feel any real discomfort, stop and come out of the posture.

Fig. 257   When the right elbow rests easily on the floor, the left is lowered, as illustrated. All previous statements regarding care and caution apply to this movement as well. When both elbows are able to rest on the floor, hold the feet as depicted.

Fig. 258   The completed posture. The top of the head rests on the floor; the hands hold the feet; the knees are together; breathe as slowly as possible. Hold for a count of 10.

To come out of the posture, reverse the order of the movements, that is, raise your head so that you are in the position of *Fig. 257;* roll onto your right elbow as in *Fig. 256* and slowly straighten up.

When you are able to perform the Extreme Backward Bend, substitute it for the less advanced Backward Bend. If performing this exercise on the toes appears too difficult, you may try it with the feet on the floor as in *Fig. 74*. This will be much easier. Remember that this is one of the most advanced Yoga postures and will come when great flexibility of the spine has been achieved.

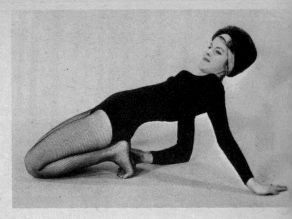

Fig. 256

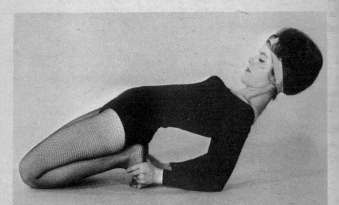

Fig. 257

Fig. 2

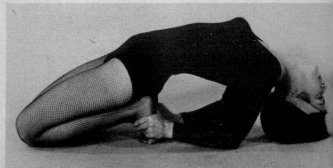

LOCKED LOTUS

Fig. 259   This is an advanced variation on the Full-Lotus, *Fig. 83*. It helps to promote great flexibility and is an intensive aid in improving the posture.

The heels must be placed high on the thighs, close in toward the groin. Reach behind your back with your left hand and attempt to grasp the toes of the left foot. Holding this position for a count of 20 will gradually permit you to reach around with your right hand and hold your right foot. You will undoubtedly have to struggle to achieve the completed posture of *Fig. 259*, but once you accomplish it the first time it becomes easy thereafter. Holding this posture for a count of 20 is excellent for your back and shoulders.

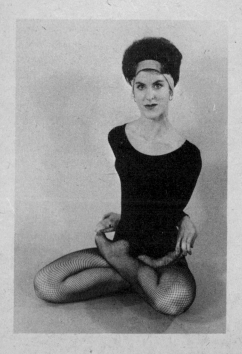

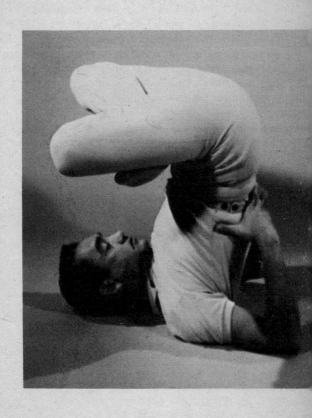

LOTUS SHOULDER STAND

Fig. 260 Assume the Full-Lotus. Lie down and swing your locked legs up as illustrated. Bring up your hands for support.

Fig. 261 Attempt to straighten the legs as illustrated.

When you are able to perform the Lotus Shoulder Stand easily, it should be held for approximately one minute of the three or more minutes suggested for the Shoulder Stand. The complete Shoulder Stand routine would then be as follows: one minute in the Lotus Shoulder Stand, straighten the legs into the vertical position for approximately two to three minutes, perform the Shoulder Stand Variations.

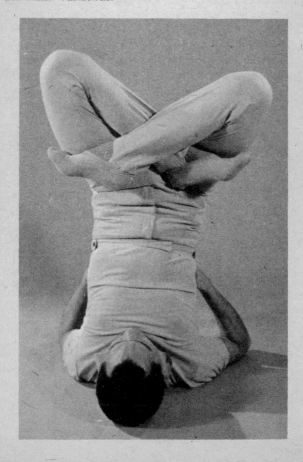

Part Six

Practice Routines;
General Information

The following chart presents a simple, concise way to use the Yoga exercises for physical fitness in a daily plan that requires approximately fifteen to twenty minutes. Four groups of exercises are used *consecutively* for daily practice. For example, on Monday you would practice Group 1; on Tuesday, Group 2; Wednesday, Group 3; Thursday, Group 4. Then on Friday you would return to Group 1, and so forth. It is important that you keep note of which group you have done on each day because if your practice is interrupted for any reason you should take up wherever you left off. For example, if you were to practice Group 1 on Monday, Group 2 on Tuesday and you were unable to practice on Wednesday, you would begin with Group 3 on Thursday. In this manner you will include all of the desired exercises in each four days of practice.

The four groups consist of exercises taken from the seven categories of Part I of this book. Each day you will be practicing one exercise from each group, with one or two minor exceptions. This will enable you to work on all areas of the organism each day. Because of the great importance of breathing and internal exercising for everyone, the Complete Breath and the Abdominal Lift are included in *each of the four groups, since they are to be performed each day*. Daily meditation is optional.

Any of the "Yoga During the Workday" exercises of Part II can be performed during the course of regular practice if desired. The Chest Expansion is always a wonderful technique for any period of practice.

The "special problem" routines must be included as the individual deems necessary. If weight control is a problem, then the four exercises indicated for this can be included in each day's practice, or perhaps every other day. If posture is the problem the two indicated techniques could probably be included daily. It is virtually impossible to give explicit directions of how to arrange the exercises for a particular problem. This depends on the time available for practice.

The housewife should perform the designated exercises in Part IV each day. After she has completed this routine of eight techniques she can perform any of the other exercises. It might be a good idea to include a few different postures from the various categories each day.

The extreme positions of Part V gradually replace the more modified positions of the other categories.

The time of the day that you practice is up to you. Fit your practice into your schedule as best you can (it would be best to exercise at the same time each day) but once you do begin try not to be interrupted. It may be convenient for you to practice half of the exercises in the morning and do the rest of the group later in the day. Remember that all of the information regarding the number of repetitions and the time for holding the extreme positions is given to you in the instructions of each exercise. You should follow this information closely until you become quite adept with the techniques, then you can add time or repetitions as you wish. Certain exercises may be exceptionally good for you and you may want to include these exercises every time you practice; this is perfectly satisfactory, but do not neglect the other exercises of the group. If any of the exercises seem to be more difficult than others, perform them cautiously and without strain, but do not neglect them. If you are serious in your practice you should eventually be able to do every one of the exercises.

THE FOUR BASIC GROUPS [*]

1.

Complete Breath (in Lotus)
Complete Breath Standing
Abdominal Lift
Leg Clasp
Toe Twist
Elbow Exercise
Preliminary Leg Pull
Cobra
Side Raise
Meditation (optional)

2.

Complete Breath
Abdominal Lift
Rishi's Posture
Shoulder Raise
Knee and Thigh Stretch
Alternate Leg Pull
Back Push-Up
Bow
Meditation (optional)

3.

Complete Breath
Abdominal Lift
Neck Twist
Full Twist
Complete Leg Pull
Backward Bend
Shoulder Stand
Locust
Meditation (optional)

4.

Complete Breath
Abdominal Lift
Arm and Leg Stretch
All Fours
Eye Exercise
Scalp Exercise
Lie Down—Sit Up
Plough
Head Stand (or Shoulder
    Stand may be substituted)
Meditation (optional)

GENERAL INFORMATION

1 For practice, choose a quiet place with a good supply of
fresh air.

2 Remove all tight and confining clothing, including belt,
watch, shoes and glasses. Actually, the less clothing, the
better.

---

[*] Exercises from other categories may be added to these basic groups
as indicated in previous discussion.

3 Use the same mat or pad for your practice each day. Do not allow it to be used for any other purpose.

4 For some exercises you will need your watch or clock, so keep it handy.

5 Keep a notebook to write down which group you are practicing on a given day and to make other notes regarding the exercises you may wish to add to your practice.

6 Do not practice for at least ninety minutes after eating. You may eat after practicing if you wish.

7 You have been given complete instructions as to the time and routines for practice.

8 The application of Yoga to special problems and the consulting of one's physician has been discussed in detail.

9 It is most important not to be distracted during practice and to place yourself in a calm, serene state of mind before you begin. The Complete Breath (the first exercise practiced each day) will help impart tranquillity.

With each day of Yoga practice you will find yourself making new advances. It is important that you understand you will be stretching and strengthening many areas of your body that have probably not been methodically exercised in many years. This may result in some minor discomforts; slight aches and pains can occur from time to time as the organism rebuilds. If you have days when you experience such minor discomforts, simply practice very easily or even temporarily discontinue the particular exercises that are causing the strain. In a day or two this uncomfortable feeling will pass and you can continue your practice. If you follow this procedure and never strain, you will find new strength and life in even the most difficult and stubborn areas of your body.

Index

EVERY YOGA FAN WILL WANT TO READ . . .

BE YOUNG WITH YOGA (89-432/$1.95)
   by Richard L. Hittleman

JOY OF LIFE THROUGH YOGA (76-736/$1.25)
   by Eugene Rawls & Eve Diskin

RENEW YOUR LIFE THROUGH YOGA (78-936/$1.50)
   by Indra Devi

YOGA FOR BEAUTY AND HEALTH (89-400/$1.95)
   by Eugene Rawls & Eve Diskin

YOGA FOR PERSONAL LIVING (89-433/$1.95)
   by Richard L. Hittleman

YOGA FOR PHYSICAL FITNESS (89-099/$1.95)
   by Richard L. Hittleman

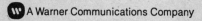 A Warner Communications Company

Please send me the books I have checked.

Enclose check or money order only, no cash please. Plus 35¢ per copy to cover postage and hanlding. N.Y. State residents add applicable sales tax.

Please allow 2 weeks for delivery.

WARNER BOOKS
P.O. Box 690
New York, N.Y. 10019

Name ....

Address ....

City .... State .... Zip ....

_____ Please send me your free mail order catalog